MAKING UNCERTAINTY

MEDICAL ANTHROPOLOGY: HEALTH, INEQUALITY, AND SOCIAL JUSTICE

Series editor: Lenore Manderson

Books in the Medical Anthropology series are concerned with social patterns of and social responses to ill health, disease, and suffering, and how social exclusion and social justice shape health and healing outcomes. The series is designed to reflect the diversity of contemporary medical anthropological research and writing, and will offer scholars a forum to publish work that showcases the theoretical sophistication, methodological soundness, and ethnographic richness of the field.

Books in the series may include studies on the organization and movement of peoples, technologies, and treatments, how inequalities pattern access to these, and how individuals, communities, and states respond to various assaults on well-being, including from illness, disaster, and violence.

For a list of all the titles in the series, please see the last page of the book.

MAKING UNCERTAINTY

Tuberculosis, Substance Use, and Pathways to Health in South Africa

ANNA VERSFELD

RUTGERS UNIVERSITY PRESS

New Brunswick, Camden, and Newark, New Jersey
London and Oxford

Rutgers University Press is a department of Rutgers, The State University of New Jersey, one of the leading public research universities in the nation. By publishing worldwide, it furthers the University's mission of dedication to excellence in teaching, scholarship, research, and clinical care.

Library of Congress Cataloging-in-Publication Data

Names: Versfeld, Anna, author.
Title: Making uncertainty : tuberculosis, substance use, and pathways to health in South Africa / Anna Versfeld.
Description: New Brunswick : Rutgers University Press, 2023. | Series: Medical anthropology | Includes bibliographical references and index.
Identifiers: LCCN 2022017020 | ISBN 9781978822474 (paperback) | ISBN 9781978822481 (cloth) | ISBN 9781978822498 (epub) | ISBN 9781978822511 (pdf)
Subjects: LCSH: Tuberculosis—Patients—Substance use—South Africa—Cape Town. | Tuberculosis—Treatment—South Africa—Cape Town. | Tuberculosis—Social aspects—South Africa—Cape Town. | Substance abuse—South Africa—Cape Town.
Classification: LCC RA644.T7 V47 2023 | DDC 362.19699/5009687355—dc23/ eng/20220715
LC record available at https://lccn.loc.gov/2022017020

A British Cataloging-in-Publication record for this book is available from the British Library.

rutgersuniversitypress.org

CONTENTS

FOREWORD

LENORE MANDERSON

The *Medical Anthropology: Health, Inequality, and Social Justice* series is concerned with the diversity of contemporary medical anthropological research and writing. The beauty of ethnography is its capacity, through storytelling, to make sense of suffering as a social experience and to set it in context. Central to our focus in this series, therefore, is the way in which social structures, political and economic systems, and ideologies shape the likelihood and impact of infections, injuries, bodily ruptures and disease, chronic conditions and disability, treatment and care, and social repair and death.

Health and illness are social facts: the circumstances of the maintenance and loss of health are always and everywhere shaped by structural, local, and global relations. Social formations and relations, culture, economy, and political organization as much as ecology shape experiences of illness, disability, and disadvantage. The authors of the monographs in this series are concerned centrally with health and illness, healing practices, and access to care, but in the different volumes, the authors highlight the importance of such differences in context as expressed and experienced at individual, household, and wider levels. Health risks and outcomes of social structure and household economy (for example, health systems factors), as well as national and global politics and economics, all shape people's lives. In their accounts of health, inequality, and social justice, the authors move across social circumstances, health conditions, geography, and their intersections and interactions to demonstrate how individuals, communities, and states manage assaults on people's health and well-being.

As medical anthropologists have long illustrated, the relationships between social context and health status are complex. In addressing these questions, the authors in this series showcase the theoretical sophistication, methodological rigor, and empirical richness of the field, while expanding a map of illness, social interaction, and institutional life to illustrate the effects of material conditions and social meanings in troubling and surprising ways. The books reflect medical anthropology as a constantly changing field of scholarship, drawing on research in such diverse contexts as residential and virtual communities, clinics, laboratories, and emergency care and public health settings; with service providers, individual healers, and households; and with social bodies, human bodies, biologies, and biographies. While medical anthropology once concentrated on systems of healing, particular diseases, and embodied experiences, today the field has expanded to include environmental disasters, war, science, technology, faith, gender-based violence, and forced migration. Curiosity about the body and its vicissitudes remains a pivot of our work, but our concerns are with the location of bodies in social life and with how social structures, temporal imperatives, and shifting exigencies shape life courses. This dynamic field reflects the ethics of the discipline to address these pressing issues of our time.

As the subtitle of the series indicates, the books center on social exclusion and inclusion, social justice and repair. The volumes in this series illustrate multiple ways in which globalization and national and local inequalities shape health experiences and outcomes across space; economic, political, and social inequalities influence the likelihood of poor health and its outcomes in different settings. At the same time, social and economic relations enable the institutionalization of poverty; they produce the unequal conditions of everyday life and work and hence, also, of who gets sick and who is most likely to survive. The books challenge readers to reflect on suffering, deficit, and despair within families and communities, while they also encourage readers to remain alert to resistance and restitution—to consider how people respond to injustices and evade the fissures that might seem to predetermine their lives.

With the twin pandemics of tuberculosis (TB) and substance use, as Anna Versfeld describes in *Making Uncertainty: Tuberculosis, Substance Use, and Pathways to Health in South Africa*, the inequalities of life circumstances directly impact on infection, treatment, care, and recovery. In this compelling account, Versfeld turns to personal circumstances and structural forces, including the pull of family members and concerns about them, and the challenges of care provision in contexts of marginalization. Experiences and affective ties converge to work against people's ability to remain inpatients for treatment for TB and diminish the likelihood of cure.

TB is curable, but it remains a leading cause of death worldwide. It is still the leading cause of death in South Africa. In 2019, 1.4 million people died of TB globally; 58,000 people died of TB in South Africa, some two thirds of whom were coinfected with HIV (SAMRC, HSRC, and NICD 2020). The majority are poor, living in conditions of deprivation in which TB thrives. The precarities of people's everyday lives are so overwhelming that hospitalization is often the only way to ensure treatment, care, and, ideally, cure. The setting for Anna Versfeld's extraordinary book is DP Marais Hospital, which operates in Cape Town. The background is the homemade shacks, lanes, and meeting places that crowd the fringes of Cape Town and the precarious spaces of shelter nearer to the central business district. For DP Marais patients, life in these settings can be chaotic. The conditions in which people survive, the combination of poverty, violence, and the limits of state interventions, gender-based violence, and the use of drugs, all contribute to a context in which people are at risk of infection with TB. Many of those admitted to DP Marais have a long history of alcohol and drug use; many are also infected and being treated for HIV. Others simply live with little support, and the uncertainties of everyday life, social exclusion, and family tension make residential care a particularly compelling option. People were admitted to the hospital for care as a way of managing their struggles to balance treatment with income generation, family care, stretched finances, and noisy, difficult lives. The hospital offers people consistency of care to effect cure.

When people with TB enter the hospital, they are often desperately sick. Their stay in DP Marias is perhaps their best chance to recover and so avoid untimely death. Those who are hospitalized receive supervised treatment for TB, and they participate in interventions for drug dependency, albeit with varying success; those who habitually use substances in the community do not necessarily cease to do so on the ward. People may also take weekend leave, or leave the hospital while still under treatment, and so may face all the problems that they were able to set aside while in the hospital. As Versfeld illustrates, people fall out of care and, lost to follow-up, their infection can return with voracity.

Here lies the frustration for health providers, including the doctors and nurses on the wards of DP Marais, who are concerned that repeated interruptions to treatment may require longer periods of hospitalization. Resentful hospital staff sometimes treat patients dismissively, occasionally subjecting them to rebuke, largely venting their own frustrations and the limits to which they can make a difference. For while health providers may see patients as morally flawed and as "failing" treatment, rather than as people who struggle to remain in the hospital to receive full treatment, they are mindful of the weight of poverty, family pressure, and other health problems. While some may direct their frustration at patients, others concede that patients' delays in initiating treatment and remaining in care are reflections of the insidiousness of life circumstances and the harms inherent in inequality.

Making Uncertainty is a brilliant ethnography of chaos and care, and of how treatment and cure are mediated by the limits of resources, structures, infrastructures, and support systems. Anna Versfeld helps us to see the constraints that affect staff and patients, and that undermine the provision of care. The background is not of individual drug and alcohol misuse, therefore, but of endemic inequality, unemployment, and the difficulties faced by the state and its institutions to allocate resources and provide health and social services. Versfeld quotes one young interlocutor—"every drug has its day." It's a cold reflection on the place of treatment for TB and on the mundaneness of substance use as a way of coping. It's a commentary too on the persistence and pervasiveness of extreme poverty, the difficulties of remaining on treatment to cure a pernicious disease.

Ultimately, systemic challenges rather than individual behaviors explain why TB persists.

REFERENCE

SAMRC (South African Medical Research Council), HSRC (Human Sciences Research Council), the NICD (National Institute for Communicable Diseases). 2020. *The First National TB Prevalence Survey, South Africa 2018. Short Report.* Cape Town: Tuberculosis Platform, South African Medical Research Council.

MAKING UNCERTAINTY

1 · RETURNERS

Dr N says that when drug users leave [the hospital] they get sick again. Then they return [to the hospital], get "clean" again, return to society, default[1] their medication, get sick again, and return again. The issue, she explains, is that on returning [to the hospital] they know how to abuse the system.

—Doctor interview, DP Marais TB Hospital, May 2014

On his first admission to the TB, Jeffrey was close to death. He had, he said, ignored his breathlessness, hacking cough, and extreme weakness until an acquaintance—fearing he would die beside him—called an ambulance. The ambulance deposited Jeffrey at a tertiary care hospital,[2] where he was diagnosed with advanced drug-sensitive pulmonary TB and sent on to DP Marais, one of the two subacute TB hospitals in Cape Town, South Africa.

In the hospital, Jeffrey (husband four times over, once a gang heavy and a convicted armed robber) was a model patient. Over a five-month period, he regained strength and health. He did not use drugs. He put flesh to bones. Nearing the end of his treatment, he was discharged from the hospital, on the basis that he had a "good family" and parents who could accommodate him. He no longer had the angularity of a s(t)ick man and was "sputum negative" (not infectious). He left promising (me, himself, and the hospital staff) he would never touch drugs again. He would be a good father to his four daughters and a submitting son to his troubled parents. He would stay with his mother and stepfather and finish his TB treatment. He would take and make this opportunity to start afresh. Different. Healthy.

Five months later, I found Jeffrey lying on a mattress pulled outside into the late afternoon sun beyond the glass doors of the locked ward where he was now resident. An arm was slung over his face to protect his eyes from the low-hanging afternoon rays. He was so very much thinner than he had been when I last saw him that for a moment, I doubted that it was him. As I peered at him, trying to ascertain whether the gaunt face was the one I knew, he opened his eyes and he sat up, "Anna!" I had barely finished greeting him when, somewhat contrite, he said, "When I got out I did everything I promised I wasn't going to do . . . now I have [multiple drug-resistant] TB." My response was similarly forthright,

"I'm afraid that's what tends to happen. . . ." Then, with an edge of cheer, Jeffrey asked, "Am I now a main character in your research?" I found myself shooting back, "Well, you are the perfect case study. . . ." And then, ashamed at my callousness, I added, "Though I would really much rather you weren't. . . ."

In his question, "Am I now a main character in your research?" Jeffrey was astutely acknowledging the dynamics of our friendly but careful and research-weighted relationship. He was well aware that his reappearance in the hospital marked him as a "returner," a patient who had been discharged apparently on the road to health but who was readmitted in the full throes of TB again. People who used substances frequently cycled in and out of the DP Marais hospital in this way. It was an immense frustration for hospital and TB clinic staff. "I hope I never see you again," was the joke one of the hospital doctors would make when a patient was being discharged. It was funny because she meant it. It was sad because it was, so often, a hope unfulfilled, especially with people who used substances.

TACKLING INTRACTABILITY THROUGH EXAMINING CO-CONSTITUTION

In 2012, I conducted a short stint of research in three TB clinics in Cape Town. Having just completed other research on people who use drugs, I was attuned to noticing the nuances of interactions with and about them. I noticed that families of patients who used substances were appealing to the health care system for protection from infectious kin, and health care workers were frustrated by, and fearful of, providing services to people who used drugs. Exploring the international literature, I found a well-established relationship between TB and substance use, more broadly (inclusive of alcohol). People who use substances face increased TB transmission rates (Oeltmann et al. 2009; Deiss, Rodwell, and Garfein 2009) due to poor living conditions and high rates of incarceration, both of which increase the chances of TB infection (World Health Organization 2008). Once infected, they are more likely to develop active TB (Friedman et al. 1987), at least partly due to the immune suppression that some substances— such as alcohol, methamphetamine, and cannabis—cause (Oeltmann et al. 2009). They also have increased chances of severe illness and drug-resistant strains of infection (Morozova, Dvoryak, and Altice 2013). The likelihood of severe infection is fostered by avoidance of health care systems or, to use public health parlance, "delayed treatment seeking" (Leonhardt et al. 1994; Oeltmann et al. 2009; Gundersen, Yimer, and Bjune 2008); increased chances of treatment interruption (or default); and decreased chances of treatment completion (Malotte, Rhodes, and Mais 1998; Leonhardt et al. 1994; Oeltmann et al. 2009; Deiss, Rodwell, and Garfein 2009). Treatment default or interruption increases the chances of TB relapse and morbidity (Cramm et al. 2010). One South African study notably showed that inhaling mandrax—a popular local neuro-suppressant narcotic (see below)—during treatment was the biggest risk factor for multiple drug-resistant (MDR) TB. The same study showed that alcohol was an important risk factor for treatment default (Holtz et al. 2006). International policy guidelines have recommendations on the intersection of TB and substance use (World Health Organization, United Nations Office on Drugs and Crime, and UNAIDS 2008; Getahun, Baddeley, and Raviglione 2013). Quotidian local experience seemed to align with the international literature, but local academic and policy arenas were notably silent.

Intrigued, I set about exploring what was happening when TB and substance use overlapped in people accessing care facilities in Cape Town. In addition to my time at DP Marais TB Hospital, which drew patients from the city and further afield in the Western Cape Province, I spent four months based in a Matrix public outpatient substance use treatment clinic in Delft, a poor residential neighborhood on the fringes of the Cape Town. As it appeared (and was presented) in the health care facilities, the dynamic interaction of TB and substance use had the makings of an intractable problem: substance use resulted in erratic lives and was linked to avoidance of the health care system and to treatment interruption. People who habitually used substances rarely stopped use, even when ill. TB required consistent treatment for an extended period—at the very least, six months. Repeated TB treatment interruption increased the chances of drug-resistant strains of TB, which, in turn, required longer treatment periods. Lack of treatment, however, meant continued illness, continued infectiousness.

In this book, I unpick the local dynamics of the knotted synergy between TB and substance use to provide depth to this surface reading of what was going on. Per capita, the TB incidence rates in South Africa are some of the highest in the world. At the time I was conducting the bulk of my research (2014), the cure rate for drug-sensitive (DS) TB was 75 percent, 10 percent lower than the success rate described by the World Health Organization (WHO) as necessary for containing the epidemic (World Health Organization 2013).[3] South Africa also had a well-established epidemic of drug-resistant TB and a growing—and panic-inducing—number of patients with the practically untreatable, extremely drug-resistant (XDR) TB (Churchyard et al. 2014). TB has been the leading cause of death since 2001. Currently, someone dies every seven minutes.[4]

Substance use rates were also frequently described as being of epidemic proportions, especially in the popular press, though the data proving this were (and remain) rather more sketchy. Epidemics are worthy of study for, to use Paul Farmer's (1992) turn of phrase, they lay bare "geographies of blame"—who is seen as responsible for poor health. And, as Didier Fassin writes, they "are moments of truth when both knowledge and power are put to the test" (2007, 32).

The confluence of epidemics (real and perceived) raises additional areas of enquiry: How, where, why, and to what extent do they meet? What happens at the epicenter of the intersection, and how do the effects ripple out?

In this approach, my work fits into a growing body of social science literature focused on the synergistic interaction between a variety of diseases and health conditions and the ways in which this is seated within social relations. Much of this literature—and increasingly literature that fits more strictly into the bio-medical field—draws on Merrill Singer's concept, "syndemics." A portmanteau of the words "synergy" and "epidemic," Singer defines the term as "the concentration and deleterious interaction of two or more diseases or other health conditions in a population" as a consequence of "social inequity and the unjust exercise of power" (2009, 226).

Syndemics draws attention to the ways in which poor social conditions foster poor health; health conditions can—as discussed above—feed off and exist within each other; and diseases cluster and co-occur in certain populations due to shared social conditions. This, as I discuss further in Chapter 3, contrasts to biomedical descriptions of diseases as discrete entities. Medical nosology, the classification of diseases, requires that a disease is sufficiently distinct from others as to fit only into one classificatory location. This is both key for how diseases are understood epistemologically and is also the basis of treatment. Medication is designed to target specific pathogens, and treatment tends to require the isolation of distinct pathogens that can be pharmacologically targeted. This particularistic, biomedical approach, however, has numerous limitations: it ignores the context in which health conditions develop within. It also does not acknowledge that health conditions can develop symbiotically or can be reliant on each other for development (in particular forms). Here, the way in which TB thrives when someone already has HIV is illustrative. Finally, as has been shown by others (Weaver and Mendenhall 2014; Engelmann and Kehr 2015), health conditions can interact synergistically to become something greater than the sum of their parts. Again, TB and HIV provide a good illustration. When they are mutually present, they tend to compound each other as a synergism develops between them.[5] Interacting diseases often result in constellations of symptoms that fit into neither original disease category. The biomedical term to describe this, "comorbidity," simply does not encapsulate these complexities.

The syndemics literature, then, I suggest, does important work in illustrating that it is impossible to cleave the social and the medical and that biomedical conceptions of diseases as discrete entities fail to provide a full picture of the ways in which health conditions interact. However, my observation is that the concept of syndemics does not do justice to the value of a social science engagement with health and illness or to lived experience. As I describe further in Chapter 3, Singer's earlier work, which builds the concept, examines the interaction of substance abuse, violence and AIDS (2000, 2006). This emphasizes how political economic relations interact dynamically in the making of poor health. However, in later work, Singer and Clair (2003) distinguish between a syndemic at a population level, described as "two or more epidemics interacting synergistically and contributing as a result to an excess *disease* load in a population," and at an individual level, where it is described as "health consequences of the *biological interactions* that occur when two or more diseases or health conditions are co-present in multiple individuals within a population" (emphasis added). Yet, as I show in Chapter 5, primary health care workers may experience drug use as their "biggest problem" in TB treatment, but this is less because drugs themselves have any innate characteristics to make people behave in particular ways and more due to the ways in which health care workers often discriminate against people who use drugs, setting up an antagonistic patient–provider relationship and undermining the goal of treatment completion. Drug use does not need to fit into the category of condition or disease to have a notable impact on people's health. The shrinking of the concept of syndemics to refer solely to biology and the emphasis on biological interactions, then, undercuts some of the concept's capacity to blur the boundaries between the social and the biomedical, and it is precisely in this blurring—the reminder that health cannot be understood outside of social context—that the term syndemics has value.

This narrowed understanding of what matters in shaping health and disease also does not do justice to the complexity of lived experience. In contrast to the ways in which primary health care providers emphasized the importance of drug use (though for the wrong reasons), senior medical staff described it as "a complicating factor." The fact that substance use might have played a role in the constitution of poor health was less important than the immediate needs of attained improved health. The doctor's framing aligned with the way that syndemics is currently framed—social life matters because it shapes the ways in which health conditions come to interact.

Beyond this, the current syndemics literature focuses on that which is generated out of, or through, the syndemic interaction being described. Yet, as I show through stories about how health and illness are constituted,[6] substance use can mask TB symptoms and shape an alternative reading of the body so that the person affected does not recognize the presence of TB despite the symptoms being well known in poor communities. Substance use can further complicate TB clinicians' diagnostic options and therefore their treatment options. Interacting health forces deepen the murk in which patients read their bodies and health care providers' work. The effect of interacting health forces demands and deserves our attention not only because of what they produce, but also because of the ways in which the obscure and obfuscate cause and effect in the constitution of the health statuses. Attention should, I suggest, linger on that which is masked as much as that which is made. Both have ramifications for health and illness. Through all of this, my work reframes the ways in which "health forces"—as all the elements that shape health experiences, understandings, and responses—"co-constitute," or set, the conditions for and build each other.

A DIVIDED COUNTRY BREEDS A DIVIDED CITY

The City of Cape Town fills a hooked finger of land that juts from the southwestern rim of South Africa. Brochures advertising the city make much of its iconic table-topped mountain and the elegant mountain range that spines the peninsula, its numerous beaches, and the winelands it extends into. But tourists flying in would be hard-pressed not to notice that is a city defined by contrasts; the mountain's green frock grays as the peninsula flattens and widens into the rest of the province. Here the scrubby land of the "Cape Flats" becomes densely overlaid with a sprawl of small, squat government-supplied houses and tightly packed informal dwellings constructed during (and since) apartheid on the sands blown, over millennia, off the coast. Understanding the construction of the city, and the history of state care and nurturance for some and oppression, dispossession, and marginalization for others, matters because it continues to impress itself on the lives and health of the populace in South Africa. It shapes who becomes sick and what they suffer from, which services they can access, and the quality of their care.

European colonists first settled in the Cape in the mid-1600s in order to provide supplies to ships passing to the riches of the East. Various waves of colonial settlement—and power struggles between settlers—came to a head at the turn of the nineteenth century, in a bitter war about whether areas of the interior (which had recently been found to be studded with diamonds and shot through with gold) should be governed by English-speaking people, or those of Dutch origin, who claimed the name "Afrikaner." In 1910, the British-led Union of South Africa was determined a self-governing dominion of the British Empire. In the new Republic, the colonial project of hierarchical, race-based social division was quietly continued. In 1948, however, the Afrikaner-led Nationalist Party came to power (riding in, partly, on the ticket of promises to enforce racial division). Election promises became reality as the Party set in motion the codification, consolidation, expansion, and enforcement of the long-established structures of white power. Two laws in this process were fundamental to the project of urban division and the construction of the Cape Flats: the Population Registration Act, No. 30, of 1950 designated every South African as belonging to a particular population group—White, Coloured, African, or Indian;[7] government officials went house to house designating individuals and families as one race or the other through individualized judgments of social class and phenotypical presentation (Posel 2001). The Group Areas Act of 1951 mapped the urban landscape into specific racially defined residential areas. Though the project was never completed in Cape Town, for the most part, people who were not classified White and who were living in the coveted prime residential areas close to the mountain were forcibly removed to poor quality housing on the sands of the Cape Flats. Some of the emptied homes and neighborhoods were bulldozed, and others were handed over to families with the "right" racial profile for the designation of the area.

Today, Cape Town has a population of four and a half million people. The twenty-five years of democracy have done little to alter the divided contours of the city, which remains cleaved along race and class lines. The Gini coefficient (indicating inequality) is a dismal 0.61 (Western Cape Government 2017). The land close to the mountain, education, assets, and opportunities are concentrated in the White population. The Cape Flats population, overwhelmingly poor, has densified as families have added generations, and rural populations, also carved out by apartheid-forced removal processes, have sought livelihoods in the city. As an economic hub, poverty rates are some of the lowest in the country, but the bar is low: over a third of people in the city are documented, in official statistics, as living below the upper bound poverty line, and 13.9 percent of households are recorded as having no income in 2016 (Western Cape Government 2016). In these conditions, both TB and substance use thrive.

Delft, where the Matrix Clinic was situated, lies on the far side of the international airport that had once marked the city boundaries. Social conditions are— for many—dire. The area is crowded, with most recent records indicating 36,000 people resident in 2.6 square kilometers (Statistics South Africa 2013). Unemployment rates are estimated to be 45 percent and many of those employed spend hours each day in gridlocked traffic that crawls the 30 kilometers up the highway toward the city center. The south of Delft includes one of the biggest blights on the record of the local municipality: Blikkiesdorp,[8] a densely populated residential area of tin shacks, which has the uniform glint of unpainted corrugated iron, constructed by the City of Cape Town almost twenty years ago as "temporary" housing. Referred to in media reports as a "dumping ground for unwanted people" (*Mail and Guardian* 2009),[9] Blikkiesdorp has now settled into permanence in the sands on which it was constructed. TB is endemic in the area—the Delft South TB clinic was the smallest of three TB treatment facilities in the neighborhood and treated approximately 800 people per month. Substance use and gang violence were also endemic. The level of violence in the area is, to some extent, illustrated by the fact that the parking bays on the street side of the clinic were always empty—avoided in case of stray bullets.

A PROBLEMATIC STATE: PATTERNING SUBSTANCE USE

The substances that fill the narratives of this book are limited and specific: alcohol, cannabis (locally referred to as dagga), methamphetamine (locally referred to as tik), and heroin (often, but not always, called nyaope). These are by no

means the only substances used and available in Cape Town. Their predomi-
nance is reflection of the ways in which substance use choices and dynamics are
clustered and concentrated in the Cape Town poor and as I describe here, pat-
terned by history.[10]

In the winelands outside Cape Town, where I grew up, weekend inebriation
among farm workers was expected, as it had been for centuries. Since the mid-
seventeenth century, farm owners, originally the Dutch colonists, provided daily
payment or rewards in the form of alcohol. This, the *dop* (tot) system, set alcohol
consumption up as one of the few sanctioned (and indeed supported) recreational activities on farms and it kept farm workers (and slaves before them)
subdued and beholden. My first piece of original research was a school project;
I designed a survey about the continued use of the *dop* system in the valley
where I lived. Determinedly, I peddled the valley rises on my bicycle, making my
way up long driveways and navigating the barking dogs to knock on solid farm-
house doors and question the often corpulent owners and managers. About a
third, if my memory serves, admitted that alcohol was still part of their weekly
pay package, though now framed as a "gift."[11] It was the early 1990s; the *dop* system had been illegal for thirty years (London 1999), but a child with a clipboard
was not threatening to admissions. Today, the provision of alcohol to workers
can result in a fine of up to a million Rand (66,000 USD) for the guilty party
(Office of the Premier of the Province of the Western Cape 2008). Payment in
the form of alcohol has left deeply rooted patterns of drinking hard and fast,
especially on the weekend, which have followed people into towns and cities. It
has also—among other things—resulted in the world's highest rates of fetal
alcohol spectrum disorder in some of the rural areas outside of Cape Town,
where almost a third of all children are affected (May et al. 2013).

Whereas alcohol use was systematically encouraged in the laboring classes,
then ostensibly discouraged by law (but condoned by turned blind eyes), cannabis use came under regulation in 1891 in the Cape, due to concerns that it was
fostering laziness, "indolence," and crime (Paterson 2009, 52) in the working
classes. This ban became a national one in 1922 when the "Customs and Excise
Duties Amendment Act prohibited the cultivation, sale, possession and use of
cannabis, cocaine and a number of opiates" (Paterson 2009, 52). In a first (and so
far only) step toward a less punitive approach to drug use, the Constitutional
Court ruled in 2018 that personal, private consumption of cannabis is not a criminal offence. However, this has not stopped police from targeting young men of
color in stop-and-search procedures and arresting them for possession (Shaun
Shelly, personal communication, September 2019). Cannabis remains the most
reported substance of use in the trends data available (Dada et al. 2019).

Even more disconcerting and insidious was the apartheid state's relationship
to the first synthetic substance to be widely used in the province: methaqualone, also known in its street form as mandrax. During the South African Truth

and Reconciliation Commission, a process of gathering narratives about the human rights violations during the latter apartheid era (1960–1994), rumors that had long circulated about covert distribution of mandrax by state operatives to men in neighborhoods designated Coloured gained some material form. Mandrax had been a central player in a chemical warfare project "Project Coast" (Gould and Folb 2002), a state-sponsored campaign of researching chemical weapons to subjugate crowds, pacify communities, and—in its ugliest form— research how to murder people in ways that would be invisible in postmortems. The story, however, had many messy threads; knotted and conflicting narratives and loose ends and assertions of clandestine mandrax distribution were not well substantiated in the scrap of contradicting versions of events (Standing 2006; Pinnock 2016). However—as Didier Fassin has argued—the rumor had power in shaping a deep mistrust of research and science that, as I turn to later, has resonated into the local HIV epidemic and, consequently, the TB epidemic. Amid the murk of misinformation, what is evident is that mandrax was originally introduced as an inexpensive sleeping tablet in the early 1970s, but it quickly came to be commonly crushed and smoked with cannabis in a broken bottleneck in what is still colloquially called a "*witpyp*" (white pipe[12]). A nervous system depressant, the result of use is deep relaxation and slumber. In communities in Cape Town where it is widely used, the term "drugs" used to be synonymous with "mandrax," indicating that it was the prevailing precursor to other chemical substances.

Around the turn of the century, broken bottlenecks lost popularity to "lollies," blown glass pipes used for smoking methamphetamine (locally referred to as "tik"). Tik's appearance was dramatic. It does not feature in the first postapartheid national strategy on drug use, the National Drug Master Plan released in 1999 (Department of Welfare, Drug Advisory Board 1999). However, by 2007, it was the most reported "drug of choice" (main drug reportedly used) in treatment centers in the Cape (Dada et al. 2015). As Andre Standing (2006) outlines, there were many reasons for this shift. The end of apartheid brought loosened border controls, reshaping the flow of illicit goods in and out of the country and—consequently—the precursors to tik, if not tik itself, became readily available. Relatively easy to make, tik manufacture became a local project, with many players. Prices dropped well below that of mandrax, making entry into the market for sellers easier, which in turn increased the number of outlets where tik was available. Increased availability fed into increased demand, the latter of which was tied to the ways in which the biochemical effects of tik—as a nervous system stimulant—interacted with postapartheid conditions in Cape Town. The years immediately postapartheid brought much-needed civil and legal freedoms, but the possibilities for crafting meaningful lives lessened as the country embarked on the structural adjustment programs required by the International Monetary Fund. In this climate, a drug that makes people feel energized and confident (though they may appear brazen or aggressive to others) found fertile ground. This appeal—as I have shown elsewhere (Versfeld, 2012a, 2012b)—was particularly strong for women who were classified Coloured living on the Cape Flats. This was a group that had previously received a modicum of support from the apartheid government, in institutional efforts to create an intermediary group between people designated White, and those designated African. For many of these women life opportunities foreclosed immediately postapartheid. Furthermore, post-mandrax-use lassitude opened women up to sexual abuse. In contrast, tik kept them awake, alert, and at least feeling like they were coping.

In 2010, I asked a group of teenage girls in Manenberg to reflect on this change. One, clear-spoken, confident, and drawing on her recent childhood, explained to me, "It's the same as the small things that come in, first it's the season for spinning-tops, then it's the season for fire crackers, that's how it is with drugs. Perhaps now it is the tik season, then the alcohol season, that's how it goes, every drug has its day." Spinning tops turn, and drug use patterns oscillate. To a large extent, it is still tik's day, which hangs on the heels of cannabis as the most reported substance at treatment centers.[13] Yet, on a meta and individual level, the "up" of tik has been countered by the increasing popularity of the "down" of heroin, which can bring the calm of sleep that tik holds at bay. Though available in South Africa since the 1980s, historically heroin was expensive, shipped in small amounts, and largely confined to a small population, largely of White males in the Johannesburg region (Haysom 2019). But it, too, is starting to have its day in South Africa, as standing international routes for Afghan-origin heroin through East Asia to Europe have closed down and the Eastern African seaboard has become the alternative funnel to the rest of the world (Haysom, Gastrow, and Shaw 2018). Increased heroin use in South Africa has been the subject of remarkably little attention, perhaps because, as others have noted (Haysom 2019; Haysom, Gastrow, and Shaw 2018), it has been mixed with an array of additional substances, which are somewhat regionally specific, and each of these combinations has had a different regional name. In 2016, when I was working with a group of people using drugs developing their skills as research-ers, the group described heroin to me as a "gutter drug": the cheapest drug there is. The group was unusual, in that almost all were injecting users, whereas most people who use heroin in the city "chase" it—inhaling the fumes released from heating the substance on a piece of foil. (The discolored or blistered lips of people who chased heroin were a tell-tale sign of use.) With time, people who smoke heroin on a regular basis tend to transition to injecting use in search of a quicker, more intense high (Haysom 2019). The most recent estimations of the number of people who inject drugs (most of which would be heroin, though some people do also inject tik) nationally, at 75,000 (Setswe et al. 2015), are in all likelihood a serious underestimation of the current situation (Haysom 2019).

TB IN TIME: THE HISTORY OF AN EPIDEMIC

In the late 1800s, South Africa was routinely advertised in European medical journals as an international destination for people suffering from consumption, as TB was previously known. The clear, arid air, especially of the interior, was described as an essential part of a "climatic cure" for the disease (Ransome 1898; Williams 1876). As the museum curator of the Kimberley Museum, once called the Kimberley Sanatorium, explained to me, the name was something of a misnomer as the institution had really been an upmarket resort, marketed to the wealthy in Europe as ideally designed and situated for the improvement of lung conditions. The Kimberley Sanatorium was the brainchild of Cecil John Rhodes, who, in a letter dated September 1895, described the institution as a "sanatorium for the treatment of persons suffering from pulmonary complaints, especially in the earlier stages, numbers of whom visit this country in search of health."

While the wealthy affected by TB could afford sanatoria, hope is everyone's currency, and people of lesser means came seeking the air, too, traveling in cramped ship berths and finding accommodation in boarding houses, ideal conditions for infection spread (Packard 1989). To some extent, then, TB was imported into the country on the European coattails of the wealthy and in the desperation of the less affluent who came seeking health, creating infection hotspots in the interior towns in which they settled. Yet more people carrying the infection came as they fled persecution in Eastern Europe, where TB rates were high.

Randall Packard's history of TB in South Africa (1989) sets out key elements of the development of TB in epidemic proportions in South Africa. As he describes, infections flourished in the multiracial urban slums, finding fertile ground in the previously unexposed (and therefore immunity-lacking) lungs of South Africans of all races, but making notable inroads into Black communities, which had previously been largely unaffected. Rapidly increasing rates of TB infection and disease in Black residents of urban slums were noted by the state officials and explained through self-serving assertions that Africans were poorly adapted to "civilized living" and lacking in knowledge of how to live in a "sanitary manner" in urban areas, making them susceptible to TB disease. While this recognizes the European origins of the disease, logic is misconstrued in that it was not acknowledged that Africans who were taking on "European" habits were most likely those who had the most contact with "European" people and, therefore, the infections they carried. The public health response (once again, both logical and twisted) played out in efforts to "educate" the Black population about the dangers of crowded living and poor nutrition, as if these were lifestyle choices. Lip service to improved conditions in poverty-stricken urban areas instead manifested as some of the first forced removals in the country; in the early 1900s, Black people—seen as reservoirs of disease—were moved to the outskirts of towns and cities to distance them from their White counterparts.

As the century settled into itself, events of the previous one came to play an increasingly important role in the spread of TB. Gold and diamond mining became centralized occupations—run by large companies, owned and managed by White men, and labored by Black men who were forced into the capitalist economy by "hut tax" (a fee on each house used as a means of generating revenue for the colonial state). Working in poorly ventilated spaces and living in cramped, poverty-stricken conditions, TB flourished in the mines and surrounding areas. And as workers went home to the rural areas, either on annual leave or because they were sick to the point of incapacitation, infection spread across the country.

The start of apartheid in 1948 dovetailed with the discovery of streptomycin as the first effective TB treatment in the same year. With this, mining companies started to provide TB treatment to affected workers, though living conditions remained dismal. The state also started to provide treatment to the severely sick in urban centers. This included the use of new treatments that came onstream over the next few decades, creating more effective treatment processes. But access to treatment and care remained patchy in urban centers and largely absent from rural areas. Limited services in rural areas were provided by nonprofit organizations, which came together under the umbrella organization, the South African National Tuberculosis Association (SANTA), in the middle of the century. TB continued to flourish, with massively discrepant rates: in the late 1970s, Africans were fifty-nine times more likely to have TB diagnosed than Whites (World Health Organization 1983).

HIV AND THE TRANSITION TO DEMOCRACY

As South Africa transitioned to democracy, the country scrambled to provide health care for all, rather than a few, rapidly increasing the amount of public health services and clinics for the majority of the population unable to afford private health care. At the same time, the country faced a wave of HIV that rolled in fast, with a remarkably steep face: in 1990, HIV seroprevalence was recorded at 0.7 percent in antenatal clinics, but by 1994, this had jumped to 7.6 percent (van der Vliet 2007). The first term of African National Congress (ANC)-led government was marked by an inconsistent and insufficient prevention-emphasis response to the growing epidemic. By the late 1990s, it was evident that a far more intensive and widespread response was required. Instead, under the stewardship of Thabo Mbeki, the government dragged its heels and then became overtly obstructionist, initially refusing to support the rollout of antiretroviral therapy (ART) or of AZT (zidovudine) to pregnant women despite the clear evidence that it prevented mother-to-child infection transmission (van der Vliet 2007).[14] Antiretroviral therapy only became available in the public health system in the

Western Cape in 1998 and then only as a the result of provincial defiance of the national government—and so earlier than in the rest of South Africa (Fassin 2007).[15] HIV lowers the immune system, effectively picking the locks and cutting the bolts of the body's defense mechanisms and leaving it vulnerable to other infections and illnesses. HIV infection not only makes TB disease more likely, it can also suppress the symptoms that are generated by the body's immune response, accelerate and exacerbate TB illness, increase the chances of forms of TB that manifest in organs other than the lungs, and ultimately increase the likelihood of TB-related mortality. Three out of every four people who die from TB are affected by HIV.

The result of government inaction was devastating; by 2005—the peak of the epidemic—almost a third of the national population was HIV seropositive and TB rates had tripled in ten years (Martinson 2009; Van Rensburg et al. 2005). These failures of the state are, as Didier Fassin (2007) writes, too easily described as simple AIDS denialism. In fact, the state response is better understood as more complex response of wariness that was seated in rumors about the state using substances framed as medication (notably mandrax) as a tool for subjugation and in memories of how Black bodies had historically been framed in the public health world as susceptible to illness because they were hypersexualized and constitutionally weak, rather than hungry, tired, stressed, and impoverished. TB was central in this historical miscasting (Packard and Epstein 1991; Packard 1989). With concerted activism, most notably from the Treatment Action Campaign, antiretroviral therapy became available to the general population, and the narrative shifted from one of skepticism to one about the right to health (Heywood 2009). At the same time, the efficacy of TB medication started, increasingly, to falter.

DOTS AND SYSTEMS OF SURVEILLANCE

Until 2014, the key approach to TB treatment in South Africa was directly observed therapy short-course (DOTS). Recommended as a global strategy by the WHO since the mid-1990s, DOTS relies on the idea that the best way to ensure someone takes their treatment, regularly and until completion, is to have them do it with someone else, ideally a health care provider, watching. The DOTS approach has faced numerous critiques. In South Africa, these have ranged from concerns about the power dynamics set up in the watcher and watched dyad (Lewin and Green 2009; Atkins et al. 2010, 2012), to purpose-unsettling arguments relating to a lack of proof of evidence that it actually improves treatment adherence (see, for example, Carroll 2013; Harper 2006, 2010), to concerns of insufficiency given the extent of the South African epidemic (Martinson 2009; Bateman 2006a; Singh, Upshur, and Padayatchi 2007).

Internationally, some enthusiasm for DOTS has waned, at least in terms of recommendations. As early as 2006, there were shifts in the WHO-led discourse away from the ideal of clinical control (watching) to patient rights and autonomy (supporting and trusting that patients do actually want to get well). This has not always translated to countries, many of which hold onto DOTS as an ideal. Technology companies have also held to this ideal, seeing marketable potential in options monitoring through a range of digital options, from "smart" pill boxes, to video-observed therapy to drone-observed therapy, to ingestible sensor monitors.

The Province of the Western Cape—often a forerunner in national approaches—quietly shifted away from national policy and toward international recommendations as early as 2005. Recognizing that TB patients, with all observation processes, did not fare better in terms of their treatment records than HIV patients who were offered far greater autonomy (along with better support), the Province stopped requiring daily observation (Atkins et al. 2012). Yet at the time of my research, the majority of TB patients in clinics, which were under the City, rather than the Province, were "directly observed" taking their treatment on a daily basis. Treatment observation periods started with patients making the daily trip to the clinic, to drink their medication under the watchful eye of the "treatment supporter." Often this was a quick visit—an arrival, a slip into a treatment room, and a rapid washdown of pills by water in a disposable cup (not unusually followed by a quick grimace) under the eye of a supervisor, who would tick the appropriate box of the monitoring card. After a period (two weeks to two months), people would graduate to in-community observation, provided by community health workers, who were (almost always) women receiving stipends to watch over a set group of TB patients. For patients with MDR TB, daily clinic visits continued until at least the first phase of treatment, during which a daily subcutaneous injection was required. This could last up to six months. Then they, too, transitioned to treatment supporters if, as I discuss in Chapter 5 they were considered "fit for DOTS."

At an individual level, DOTS seeks to ensure that individuals take their treatment consistently and complete their medication course. On a broader level, the aim is control of the level of TB in the population. Despite DOTS, South Africa was not, however, attaining the goal of 85 percent cure. The 2014 WHO report indicated that cure rates were 75 percent, 10 percent lower than required to keep the epidemic in check.

GROWING RESISTANCE

In 2006 and 2007, journal articles and titles about TB started to read like tabloid headlines:

"Living the TB resistance nightmare" (Bateman 2006a)
"'One shot' to kill MDR TB—or risk patient death" (Bateman 2007)
"XDR-TB in South Africa—no time for denial or complacency" (Singh, Upshur, and Padayatchi 2007)

The drama of these headlines (and the content of the articles) was precipitated by the detection, in 2005, of an outbreak of TB that was resistant to every form of treatment used in a state hospital in a small town, Tugela Ferry, in the province of KwaZulu-Natal. By 2006, 200 patients had been diagnosed with this terrifyingly robust strain of TB, contracted through nosocomial (in-hospital) spread, and the death rate was 85 percent (Bateman 2015).

This was the worst culmination of decades of drug-resistant TB quietly developing. Bacilli are quick to transmute, especially when targeted with only one medication. Streptomycin, as a single medication, was of limited effect until other drugs were discovered, and patients could be provided with a cocktail of drugs. Treatment periods remained a lengthy eighteen to twenty-four months until the 1960s, when the discovery of rifampicin allowed this to be shortened to a standard six months. This has slowed, but not halted, the development of drug resistance, which still emerges with "intermittent, or poorly conceived" (Farmer 1997, 348) treatment.[16]

Forms of TB are now stratified in terms of their resistance to the commonly used medications. TB strains that respond to the first two lines of treatment are now referred to as "drug-sensitive" TB. Multiple drug-resistant TB—strains that are unresponsive to at least the two main drugs currently used in TB treatment (usually rifampicin and isoniazid)—has been recognized and treated in Cape Town since the 1980s. Extensively drug-resistant TB is, like MDR TB, resistant to at least the first two lines of treatment as well as an additional set of drugs usually turned to when these usually fail (fluoroquinolones and one of the three injectable TB drugs).[17] XDR TB has been recognized in South Africa since the start of the 1990s.

With increasing resistance, treatment periods have become elastic; for drug-sensitive TB, the mandated minimum treatment period in 2014 was still six to eight months; for MDR TB, the minimum period was eighteen months; and for XDR TB, the minimum was two years. Mounting resistance brought with it an increasing barrage of toxic medication and diminishing chances of cure. In 2014, the average newly "initiated" (started on treatment) MDR patient was swallowing approximately twenty-seven tablets per day and receiving a painful daily injection into the buttocks muscle, often uncushioned by fat. This was over and above any other medication for HIV, high blood pressure, diabetes, or any other medication that might have been required.

Though injections were discontinued after two months, treatment continued for a full eighteen months.[18] Deafness was a common side effect. XDR patients took roughly the same amount of medication, for two years, though the drug combinations differed. According to WHO figures from the time, approximately three-quarters of people with drug-sensitive TB were being treated "to cure,"[19] and this dropped to less than half for MDR TB and a dismal 12 percent for XDR TB (World Health Organization 2013). Positive changes, have, however, since occurred. Bedaquiline, a new drug for drug-resistant TB, became part of the national treatment process in March 2015, has resulted in reduced treatment periods and the cessation of use of injectables for the majority of people affected, and dramatically improved treatment outcomes (Schnippel et al. 2018).

FACILITY BASES

Sjaak van der Geest and Kaja Finkler argue that hospitals are particularly useful vantage points for ethnographic enquiry because they "reflect and reinforce dominant social and cultural processes of a given society" (2004, 1996). DP Marais is no exception to this. Through the remote-controlled gates—opened and closed by a security guard—the front gable on the single-story dusty-pale yellow building of a bygone era reads:

"Princess Alice Orthopaedic Hospital"

The relief lettering references the state-run recuperation facility founded in 1933 (Louw 1979).[20] Large rooms with blue-tiled swimming pools—now empty, defunct, and locked—once provided the place for physical rehabilitation, largely for children recovering from polio and adults recovering from orthopedic surgery. Need for the facility waned with the near eradication of polio, and Princess Alice was closed down in the early 1990s, one of the many institutions that shut its doors under the auspices of rationalization as the country prepared for political and social reform.

For almost ten years, the building sat empty, until it was refurbished and occupied by DP Marais, a SANTA-supported TB rehabilitation institution founded in the early 1980s that had outgrown its previous premises. Despite having being designed for a different time and purpose, the building is relatively well configured for TB treatment. Long passages form wings that stretch out in all directions, with wards feathering off the ends. The passages are well lit and aerated by large windows and glass doors. These provide adequate light and airflow to minimize the risk of infection for staff and visitors, or between patients with different strains of TB.[21] Multiple courtyards and outside areas are available for patients to find a quiet (if not private) space, meet with family members, or simply breathe air that is not weighed down by illness or astringent with the sharp sterility of disinfectant.

The hospital came under state stewardship ten years later, but in 2014, there were still a number of staff members who had worked for SANTA and who remembered the early days of DP Marais inhabiting the Princess Alice building. They spoke of it warmly as a well-stocked institution. There were bustling and productive rooms for sewing, wood-, basket-, and metalwork. The metal medicine boxes—made in the hundreds and originally carried around by the first community care workers distributing antiretroviral (ARV) therapy in the HIV epidemic—were made by patients in the DP Marais metalwork workshop.

Two doctors in the new DP Marais hospital saw to the needs of all the patients, who, for the most part, were not desperately ill. The disease orientation of the hospital had changed, but the purpose of recuperation (rather than treatment) remained. But that has all changed. Over the past two decades, the needs of treatment shifted as the landscape of TB in Cape Town has been swept by the two (still swelling) waves of change of HIV and drug-resistant TB. HIV treatment has become integral to the hospital's work. In 2008, ARVs started to be routinely distributed to HIV-positive patients. Having HIV is more likely than not in hospital patients—data collected for this research indicated 68 percent HIV seroprevalence in 2014.[22] Whereas responding to HIV required integrating it into the everyday of care provision in all the wards, treating drug resistance is a matter of having appropriate spaces of segregation, to ensure that patients with resistant strains are not passing these on to those who do not have these same strains. In 2006, the hospital opened a separate ward for men with MDR TB (women with MDR are still managed at the other city TB hospital). The ward is separated from the rest of the hospital by a metal gate. The yard area is fenced off from the rest of the hospital grounds. Patients of this ward—marked by the flimsy paper masks they were obliged to wear when anywhere else in the hospital—only left this gated area when they were going somewhere specific. They could not join in hospital events and had their own, dedicated rooms for workshops and events.

By 2014, the basket- and metalwork rooms, like the old swimming pools, ceased to be used; the corridors were locked and the rooms strewn with feathers and bird droppings. The majority of patients were simply too sick to be up and about, let alone actively making things. It was not unusual for me to have to edge my way around a hearse pulled up to the main door if I arrived early in the morning. Not that everyone in the hospital was deathly, or even dangerously, ill. The four wards for men and two for women with drug-sensitive TB were roughly stratified by level of illness, ranging from those with "ambulant" patients (who were well enough to be up and about) where the designated doctor did rounds weekly and nurse oversight was limited, to those with acutely sick patients that had constant nurse oversight and regular doctors' rounds.

Nor should the closed passages and simple, sometimes broken, hospital infrastructure be interpreted to be indicative of the quality of the biomedical care. DP Marais is in an urban center; it was not a hospital on the margins, where "improvization" (Livingston 2012) and "routinized uncertainty" (Street 2014) characterized daily care as a result of limited or broken diagnostic and treatment resources, though this has been described in rural settings in South Africa (Gaede 2016). Advanced diagnostic procedures were not available in hospital, but they could be obtained, even if getting them done timeously often required personal negotiation with staff at tertiary hospitals.

POSITIONING AND APPROACH

My specific vantage on processes within the hospital (and therefore the broader world, if we are to take van der Geest and Finkler seriously) came from the room that I was allocated to keep my possessions, conduct interviews, and write up my research notes. It was furnished with a desk, a hospital bed, an examination light, some cupboards, and a basin. A disinfectant dispenser was positioned above the basin and, slapped by the curtains whenever the wind blew, it would release a pungent spray, a continual reminder of the presence of infectious disease and the need to avoid it.

A sign on "my" door of the room incorrectly designated me "DOCTOR." This was a title that I—even without the help of the sign on the door—was frequently, and much to my discomfort, assumed to possess. I could disavow the title, but there was no denying that, in the racially coded world Capetonians inhabit, the pallor of my (white) skin automatically signaled privilege. This, coupled with the fact that I was studying for an advanced degree, imbued a certain authority with or without a white coat. Moreover, in an exceedingly hierarchical structure, I was on a first-name basis with most of the doctors. For patients—and even some staff—this positioned me in particular ways: I was potentially a resource who could assist with a cause (attaining doctors' attention, for example). I was also potentially a threat, for, if I was aware of sensitive information—such as who was using drugs while in the hospital—and I did not maintain confidentiality, I might harm their cause.

In this context, forging relationships with patients in relation to the sensitive subject of substance use that—as I describe in Chapters 5 and 6—could easily cause patients to be discharged from the hospital, was somewhat challenging. I was also always aware of the extreme limits of privacy the hospital offered, especially during daytime hours. For the very sick, this was limited to a toilet cubical, a bathroom, and the small bubble of air that could be made in bed by a blanket pulled up over a head. I was uncomfortable spending extended time in the wards where patients could not easily escape my view and so I avoided it. Nor did I spend much time at the hospital outside of work hours, when patients had the relief of less watching eyes that came with reduced staff numbers.[23]

At the same time, I did form some robust relationships with some patients. This was partly because the location of my writeup room proved a useful one. It sat at the elbow of two corridors. One, called "the clinic," housed the pharmacy and the offices of the HIV nurse, the admissions clerk, one permanent doctor, and, each year, the new community service doctor. The other ran echoingly past the patients' records room (double locked and lined with manila folders), the social worker and auxiliary social workers' offices, the entrance to the capacious hall, the doors to Ward 4 (for men with drug-sensitive TB), the locked passage leading to defunct pools, and the occupational therapy wing. It ended in the gates to Ward 5, the ward for men with MDR TB, though another right turn, out of view, would take one along to more wards. If I left my door open as I sat writing up notes, which I did more often than not, I was visible to all who walked up the long passage. Throughout my stay, my tapping presence became an invitation to chat for a growing body of patients—many of whom were consumed by boredom—and staff alike. It was here that many of the conversations that provided the most insight into patient lives and hospital dynamics occurred. Relationships with staff in the hospital were—for the most part—easier to develop than those with patients. Eight months allowed enough time for relationships to develop, especially as I, increasingly, came to play the role of an engaged anthropologist, working alongside staff to reshape the response to substance use.

The Delft South clinic incorporated a baby clinic, a sexual and reproductive health clinic, and an HIV clinic. It had a TB clinic that tested and treated approximately 800 people per month. And, importantly, there was a Matrix clinic located in a separate prefabricated structure on the clinic grounds. Based on a (patented) American system for treating stimulant users, the Matrix largely operated through what Summerson Carr (2010) calls "the talking cure." In this, seeking abstinence is reliant on the client adopting and expressing narratives of acceptance, repentance, and change. Ways of talking deemed appropriate were so inculcated in clients who had been attending the center for a while that they pervaded all interactions. At every conversational turn, I found the logic of the treatment program. I could not get past the sense that people entering the building were playing the role of "good client," a role in which the scripts were learnt, repeated, and monitored by staff and clients alike.[24] I, too, learnt to espouse aspects of them in my daily activities in the staff team. Looking back at research notes, I see—to my own disquiet—how I, though uncomfortable with what I saw as a performance, myself became an adept performer, habitually using the terms of phrase at home in the clinic. While the Matrix features less than the hospital in this account, it provided some important insights. The confessional impulses encouraged by "the talking cure" created spaces for talking and laughing about the ways in which the participants had sought to dupe health care staff during "active" [drug-using] days. This gave me insight into the ways in which patients responded to the health care system's requirements of abstinence. I also had important conversations with the few clients who either had TB symptoms or who were on TB medication. In these conversations, we were able to break out of the expected facility narratives to gauge the fear and frustrations of trying to navigate the different public health structures for treating TB and substance use, respectively. These provide important windows into the intersections of TB and substance use outside of inpatient treatment.

In both these sites, I tacked back and forth between the classic ethnographic method of participant observation and gathering of information that could be enumerated, stretched out across spreadsheets, and turned into percentages.

Despite using these numbers as a backbone for some of the arguments in this book, my method was primarily ethnographic. I sought to attend to the meaning in gestures, in turns of phrase, carefully positioned silences, engagements, and refusals to engage. I took conversations seriously, even casual ones. I recognized that I was not the only person in any given interaction with an agenda and that sometimes there was simply no way for me to know where and how I sat in relation to other people's needs and plans. I was cognizant of the fact that what I learned was as much based on the relationships I built (or did not build) as it was about what I was trying to find. My findings were also related to my location and positioning—in place, history, and imagination. These differed greatly between the sites. This work was built on the experience of setting up and running a youth development organization in multiple neighborhoods across the city, and the research I conducted for my master's degree, in which I examined youth and drug use in one of the most socially fraught areas of the city, Manenberg. It has also been followed by the past five years of working in research and project implementation related to infectious diseases and drug use in the city. Stories from these times—and others from years before—seep into the book.

The approach I have come to in relation to substance use (though did not start with, as I detail in the closing chapter) is one of harm reduction. Harm reduction is not an explanatory framework, but rather an approach for policy and practice that focuses on reducing the harms of drug use, without judgment attached to the fact of use (Inciardi and Harrison 1999). Harm reduction interventions span from the provision of sterile needle equipment for people who inject drugs in order to avoid the transmission of bloodborne viruses, to the decriminalization of drug use, in order to move away from punitive approaches, such as arrest and incarceration of people who use drugs. I elaborate more on this in the chapter that follows.

COMING TO TERMS

In presenting this work, I am challenged by the inflexibility of some terms and the inadequacy of others. As described above, a key issue at play is that we do not have the words available for discussing something that affects health but is not necessarily a disease or a condition. The problem of this absence is well illustrated by substance use. How, when, and if drug use moves from being considered a behavior to being considered a condition, a dependence, or a disease is hotly contested.[25] And in truth, it does not necessarily need to reach any of these classifications to have very real ramifications for the ways in which people read their bodies and the way in which they are treated by the health care system. Noting this, I use "health forces" as a broader term that refers to factors, circumstances, and contexts that shape health experiences understandings and responses in ways that impact health states and outcomes.

But my challenges stretched beyond this. As I attempted to unpack the meanings and implications of commonly used words (drug, substance, use, abuse, dependence, addict, addiction, disorder, problem, and so on), I was continually stymied by the difficulties of saying what I want to say in a succinct, precise enough way without being ambushed by the various discursive frameworks to which the term is linked (see Chapter 2). I therefore outline terms I employ below, indicating where these differ from local legislation and policy and common usage.

I use the term "substances" to include alcohol and drugs. The prior, as a distinct chemical compound present in any alcoholic drink, is possibly the only dispassionately defined term I have had at my disposal. Defining "drugs" is singularly more challenging. The South African "Drugs and Drug Trafficking Act 140" (1992) rather hazily defines a drug as "any dependence-producing substance, any dangerous dependence-producing substance or any undesirable dependence-producing substance." The difficulty here is that the line between drug and medication is often only writ in name, dosage, and whether there is permission by a medical authority for use, rather than in the difference of a chemical compound.[26] It does not account for the ways in which social acceptability shapes which substances are regarded as problematic and which not. (Beyond alcohol and cigarettes, substances such as sugar and coffee may also be dependence producing but are not in any official way classified as drugs.) In order to clarify these blurry boundaries circumscribing what constitutes a "drug," the word "illicit"—meaning illegal—is often used as a precursor. Given that legal frameworks are themselves socially informed, this only further draws us into a self-referential cycle. Thus, when I employ the term "drug," which I do when I am referring to specifically psychoactive substances other than alcohol, I do so with a full recognition of the messy implications.

For my own analysis, I do not, however, employ the term "abuse," though it is commonly used in the international literature and South African policy and practice. This is partly due to my discomfort at the aspersions it casts on people who use substances. (Can one "abuse" anything and not be found morally wanting?) It is also because there is an illogical but socially accepted slippage between these terms for some substances but not others; any heroin use is quickly labeled abuse, whereas alcohol use generally is seen to require a measured assessment for the same classification. I am, moreover, in no position to make defining judgments as to the nature of the use by the people I have worked with, nor do I have any need to do so. My interest lies in the effect of the use on everyday life, relationships, health, and care. As I show, this is shaped as much by a combination of social and moral perspectives about drug use as it is by the physiological effects, and the former is not necessarily related to the quantity or patterns of drug used. I therefore do not try to ascertain a dividing line between the act of use and abuse, harmful use or problematic use. Nor do I seek to define people as having an "addiction," "disorder," or "dependence."

I employ "use" (without precursors), for any instances, singular or multiple, of imbibing substances in any manner. I employ "habitual use" when the user is described as—or describes themselves—as having a rhythm of regular use. I employ the phrase "disruptive substance use" to substance use that is described as interplaying with the requirements of TB medication and care provision to result in treatment interruption or default. I use "person affected by TB" for anyone who has, or has had, active TB, reserving "patient" for those who are, or have been, actively engaged in the health care system (even if erratically), though this abrades with activist voices that push against the label of patient. I use it because it highlights that position of "the patient" as a *category of thought*" (Meyers 2013, 17), meaning that health care providers and patients have particular (and sometimes contrasting) notions of what a patient is.

Where I use the term "addiction," it is in reference to participants to describe a state of being in which drugs are craved. However, I do so sparingly and only when it is used in self-description, unless I am discussing literature where it forms an analytical basis.[27] Finally, despite my rejection of the terms described above, there are instances in the text where they appear because I use them when I am quoting a conversation or text in which they have been employed. These complex descriptions take on ethnographic specificity in the text that follows in ways that make the reasons for my decisions clearer.

QUIET PRESENCES

My focus on the dynamic interaction between TB and substance use is illustrative, rather than unique. I could equally have examined TB or substance use and mental health, diabetes, stigma, social isolation, gender, malnutrition, race, or any number of other possible, common, co-constituting health forces. Each of these health forces makes an appearance in this ethnography, though none is central to my presentation. Race, however, which has already featured in this chapter, deems more of a mention, for it continues to be pivotal in shaping life and care.

On walking into the women's ward at DP Marais one sunny morning, a new patient, who had not seen me before, asked me if I was there to visit my mother. Initially, I was taken aback by this question, not seeing why this was—rather than the fact that I was conducting work of some sort or other—her first assumption. But then I realized she meant another newly arrived patient who, jarringly thin, with one iris cataract-white and the other a milky blue and matted gray hair, struck me as looking as close to death as I had ever seen a walking person. Our assumed relationship was based on a key similarity—shared Whiteness. The racial schisms of the city and country were such that patients in the hospital were almost all "Black" or "Coloured." In my time at DP Marais, I saw but a handful White patients, if that. The woman, thought to be my mother, used heroin. She slipped out of the hospital, "absconding" a few days after her arrival. The next time I saw her, she was requesting money at a traffic light close to my home, no longer taking her TB medication. A few days later, I heard from hospital staff that she had died. In the Matrix Clinic—situated in a neighborhood populated almost exclusively by people of color—I did not see not one White person.[28] The reason for this demographic patterning in the facilities is partly, as I have shown in this chapter, that both TB and the use of particular substances in habitual ways are concentrated in conditions of poverty and in Cape Town, and given both apartheid and neoliberalism's structural effects in South Africa, people of color are far more likely to be poor. Wealth and corresponding access to resources buffers people somewhat against the likelihood of TB infection and disease. It also enables people to access sophisticated private health care when they are sick and increases the chances that their conditions will be optimal for completing treatment. The lower likelihood of TB disease in White people is such that I have heard numerous stories of private health care providers not recognizing TB illness in their White patients despite the overt presence of all the symptoms as doctors' diagnosis capacities are undercut by their assumptions and expectations of who is at risk. Cape Town is divided in our imagination perhaps even more than it is in reality.

THE SHAPE OF IT

This opening chapter has served to ground the reader as to my position, approach, and the history I write into. In the next chapter, Chapter 2, I take up global and domestic health policies related to substance use, reflecting on the power, or lack thereof, of international discourses. Drawing on my ethnographic work, I show that international recommendations about eschewing moral judgment and moving toward practical, patient-centered care appear to be enacted in the hospital, but in fact, "tricks of terminology" inserted into policy documents reframe international ideas about harm reduction into moralistic discourses. This chapter, then, illustrates what I call the "stickiness of moral opinion"—the enduring way in which haunting moral judgments that cast substance use as a consequence of individual moral weakness shape public health care responses and undermine South African efforts at curing TB.

Drawing on life pathways of patients in DP Marais, Chapter 3 demonstrates how and why TB and substance use come to be mutually present and compounding and their symptoms mutually occluding or masking. It shows how this makes it difficult for patients to recognize their ill health and for health care providers to diagnose and treat. I develop the concepts of "health forces" and "co-constitution" as means to describe the complex ways in which bacteria and behavior intersect in human bodies and social worlds. I show that without adequate theorization of how health forces interact and mask each other, patient care is deficient.

Chapter 4 presents a folder review I conducted in DP Marais, which demonstrates the high proportion of patients in DP Marais who were using substances when they became ill (and perhaps also afterward). This is done through a reflexive ethnography of enumeration. Building on anthropological examinations of counting and measurement in global health, it criticizes the idea that numbers are neutral representations of reality. Through close reading of patient files, I explore the regimes of enumeration in operation in the hospital, showing the multiple layers of interpretation (by patients, staff, and me) that went into the construction of what I call "figure facts." Figure facts are numbers that are easy to grasp, neatly provide proof of an issue at hand, and therefore circulate easily, galvanizing action in ways that narrative evidence rarely does. I show how reading figures in relation to ethnographic insights—a process I call "strategic knowing"—helps us to arrive at "likely truths" as information most relevant for understanding the situation.

Chapter 5 goes on to show how DP Marais is situated in the greater health and social care system and how this has resulted in the high number of people using substances in the hospital. I show how primary health care providers are incentivized to send people who use substances to DP Marais for their own reporting purposes, how families and households appeal for state protection when they feel at risk from someone who is (potentially) infectious, and how individuals themselves may request admission when they see admission as their best available option. The result is that the hospital is situated in a very particular way in relation to the TB substance use co-constitution and to people who use drugs and their families.

I build on this in Chapter 6, where I develop current theories of care by illustrating that the targets of care may not be the people in the health care system per se but are also the people imagined to be at risk of infection. A prevailing discourse in South Africa is that state institutions fail to care adequately for patients. My research demonstrates that the question of which patients are imagined needs to be taken into account: people receiving treatment in institutions are only one part, albeit the more visible part, of a larger imaginary of need and intervention. I further illustrate how, through setting up a binary between (ab)use and abstinence, the conditions for failure and future treatment interruption were set in the hospital. By using ethnographic observations to recast the "problem" of the relation between substance use and treatment adherence, I show how solutions can be developed to what appear to be intractable problems.

Chapter 7 brings new insights to debates about confinement for drug-resistant TB and rights-based emphases on decentralized care provision. Through close attention to how patients feel about their impending discharges and departures from institutions, I demonstrate that, in a context of inequality, hospitalization can offer some patients much-needed respite from the precarity of their everyday lives. Time spent in the hospital, even when this is overtly or implicitly restrictive of movement, may be valued as time to "catching breath" and can be desired and orchestrated by patients. Blanket critiques of centralized care provision disregard the very important role restricted respite might play in TB patients' lives.

In the concluding chapter, Chapter 8, I describe the change, halting but real, in some staff members at the hospital. I document their shift away from morally infused conceptions of substance use as inherently wrong, toward recognition of substance use as a response to social marginalization. The result was new, more empathic approaches to patients who used substances. The data make a strong case for "anthropology in action."

2 · THE STICKINESS OF MORAL OPINION

There are problems that need urgent attention.... Among these, the traffic in narcotics and drug abuse need the most serious and urgent attention.... There can be no argument about the need to take urgent, visible, and effective measures to eradicate these problems.

—President Nelson Mandela,
First Presidential Address, 1994

ARE WE READY YET?

The scenes were of another world: hundreds upon hundreds of people sleeping intimately close on the ledges of old railway tunnels, under bypasses hidden by thick bush, and in the halls of decrepit buildings turned into mazes by blankets hung to provide visual privacy. My access to these places came with my implementing an evaluation of a project that provided outreach health services to people who injected drugs in three South African cities.[1] Project staff swapped used needles for sterile ones, dressed wounds, shared casual conversation and jokes, and—perhaps most important—acknowledged that the people they were interacting with were worthy of care. My very last stop in evaluation was a focus group with "stakeholders"—nongovernmental organization (NGO)–sector and government department representatives—to assess their experiences and opinions of the project. I was out of my depth before we had even started.

Officer P, a law enforcement official, shot off his first volley just after he had shaken my hand, before he had even taken a seat: "I'm asking you this: Are we ready for this yet?" Where, he wanted to know, was the evidence that harm reduction worked in the local context? While it might be proven to work in Europe, he argued, "our drug abusers" were of a different ilk and would misuse the situation. In light of this, he suggested, the project was simply promoting drug use and would do more harm than good.

Trying to hold equilibrium in the room, I deflected this opening salvo by providing a noncommittal response and turning to greet other arrivals. But the first person to introduce herself, a representative from the Department of Social Development, thwarted my plan of a gradual buildup to difficult conversations, by describing her misgivings about the project while we were still on introductions. She explained that the Provincial Drug Master Plan, a document that outlined the provincial implementation of the National Drug Master Plan (2013–2017), defined harm reduction as "preventing further use to the user through detox and rehabilitation." She indicated (to the great interest of the law enforcement officials present) that the organization was not registered as a "drug abuse treatment center" in terms of the defining local law, the Prevention of Substance Abuse Act of 2008. The project's provision of services to "drug abusers" was therefore illegal. Any hopes I had of guiding the conversation to less torrid areas were quashed as the state representatives, most of whom I had never met before, melded into a confrontational coalition and demanded that I provide answers on behalf of the project I was evaluating. My efforts to persuade them that I was in no such position fell upon deaf ears. The position Officer P had expressed at the beginning took solid purchase in the group: "our drugs abusers" were not sophisticated or educated enough to be able to make good use of harm reduction services.[2] Context and assumed local particularities were roughly wielded to justify withholding health services from people who use drugs. As a government representative had muttered, during another stakeholder discussion in the same evaluation, "They're going to die, anyway. . . ."

In this chapter, I explore some of the themes evident in the meeting: the lack of information and education about substance use in South Africa, the rejection or recasting of international evidence, and the continued representation of people who use substances as miscreants unworthy of care. I examine elements of the National Drug Master Plan (NDMP), the key South African drug policy document, and compare and contrast local and international TB policy related to people who use drugs. Through this I illustrate what I call the "stickiness" of moral opinion—the extent to which moral perspectives can make local policy and practice impervious to challenging and contradictory evidence.

SIGNS OF SUBSTANCE USE: HOW LITTLE IS KNOWN

In March 2014, billboards started appearing around Cape Town. Each featured a prominent local figure—the mayor, a radio personality, and a rugby player—and each had the same format: a plain background, a serious portrait of the featured personality staring straight at the camera, and a tagline that varied only by the name. "My name's Patricia De Lille and I have a drug problem. I don't use them, but they still affect me" said the billboard featuring the mayor, who was leading the initiative.

The billboards were responding to a moral panic brewing elsewhere in the media, where drug use was being described as "spiralling out of control" (Watermeyer 2013), a "crisis" (Jooste 2011), and an "epidemic" (Bateman 2006b). The panic was unsubstantiated; there is no accurate way of measuring levels of drug use. Best estimates indicate that 67,000 people were injecting drugs in South Africa at the time (Petersen et al. 2013). There are no substantiated estimates of the actual number of all those injecting, sniffing, and smoking drugs. A notional sense comes from police "busts," but in truth, these data are more illustrative of police performance (in all senses of the word), or lack thereof, than of levels of substance use. The extent of this notional sense was already evident in 2010 when I was conducting fieldwork in Manenberg, a disadvantaged neighborhood in Cape Town renowned for drug use and trade. In the building next to the community center where I was based, a well-known dealer was frequently besieged by siren-wailing, blue light–flashing police vehicles. No drugs were ever found, but none of the locals were surprised. It was common knowledge that raids were preceded by a tipoff, which gave just enough time for the elderly great-grandmother to stash the supplies in her underwear and take her place on her favorite chair in the living room. She would then sit regally, chatting casually to the police as they ineffectively turned the house (but not her) upside down.

Statistics from treatment centers provide another source of proxy data for who is using what substances, but these are skewed by which treatment centers are included in the count, who attends these, and why. Cape Town has a thriving private treatment center industry: a Google search reveals an astonishing array of facilities with blue swimming pools, plush furniture, and people lounging in lush gardens. These centers provide a "luxury," "world-class" service to an international clientele. In the same way that South Africa is a "surgeon and safari" destination—a place where relatively inexpensive plastic surgery is followed up with a safari trip while the nips and tucks heal—these facilities provide a quality service for wealthy foreigners seeking change (that is, as good as a holiday) and privacy.[3] One website neatly reveals the expected origins of the clientele by informing prospective clients they will not need a visa to enter the country, because "people coming from Europe or the United Kingdom do not need a visa to visit South Africa."[4] Costing up to $3,500 a month, these facilities are well outside the stretch of the average South African's pocket even if, as one center website claims, "you cannot put a price on your life, or the life of your loved ones." However, these facilities do offer quality and "value for money" for American or European consumers working from a stronger currency. In doing so, they bend the statistics away from the curve that illustrates local drug use.

On the other hand, centers such as the Matrix clinics are funded (to varying degrees) by South Africa's National Department of Social Development. These are free or of low cost to attend, reducing barriers to entry. But their figures also suffer sampling errors. The number of people using substances far exceeds the number of people attending treatment centers, and the available information does not reveal who does not go. Women, in particular, are hesitant to reveal themselves as using substances due to the more extreme stigma they suffer. Attendance is also not necessarily an act of free will. In cases of minor drug-related

offences (such as, until recently, possession of small amounts of cannabis), attendance may be court ordered or required by social workers where child abuse
and/or neglect is suspected or documented alongside drug use. Of all the adult
women newly arriving at the Delft South Matrix clinic over a one-month period
in late 2014, over a third (7/26) had referral letters indicating that their program
inclusion was a prerequisite for being allowed to keep (or regain) the right to
care for their children. No men had the same threats attached to their referrals,
revealing the reality of everyday gender discrimination.[5]

The unregistered treatment centers that operate outside of official systems and
avoid surveillance add to the difficulty of assuming that the data are representative. These facilities tend to come to attention only when there are complaints
(or deaths), and how many there are is anybody's guess. At best, then, treatment
centers provide oblique indications of use trends (Pasche and Myers 2012), but
they are the best to hand. What this means is that while we do have a good sense of
what substances are being used, we do not have any accurate sense of who is using
substances, or to what extent. Even less is known about the intimate lives, needs,
and choices of people who use drugs, because to know about this means that
people who use drugs need to be regarded as sensible, knowledgeable, and holding
worthy opinions.

The billboards, do not, however, seem to have been developed in order to
make people who use drugs seem less other. City spokesperson assertions were
that the campaign aimed at encouraging people to access treatment, but the
fact that the images included no contact information made this an unconvincing
argument. For those living in poorer areas, the ubiquitous, quotidian nature of
drug use does not need to be driven home by statistics or billboards. In Manenberg, a group of teenage boys drew me maps that marked out the houses where
drugs were sold in the two-kilometer square area where they moved freely—
there were eleven such houses. And on an afternoon before a "graduation cere-
mony" for those who had completed the Matrix Programme in Delft, I drove
one young woman, Geraldine, across a few neighborhoods to her grandparents'
house to fetch a dress to wear the next day. As we drove, she pointed out the
places one could buy drugs: there, and there, and there and there, there.…
When we reached her grandparents' house, I waited in the car while she went
inside. I watched as a steady stream of people came and went out of her grandparents' house. Those departing would tuck small see-through plastic packets
into their pockets or elsewhere on their bodies. The trade in substance use was
so common—and clearly so unregulated—that people's efforts to hide their
acquisitions were minimal—and Geraldine's struggles were put in context.

The billboards did, however, provide an opportunity for pithy political comment. A number of those featuring the mayor had the words "The city that works
for a few" stenciled over her face—a word play on the City's logo, "The City that
works for you"—in reference to the failures of the City management to decrease

inequality. People living in the craft beer and gin-sipping leafy suburbs were, and still are, more sheltered from these everyday realities, but crime is easily and quickly linked to drug use in casual conversation. (Disconcertingly, no good dinner party seems complete without a crime story or three.) This easy linkage is supported by the national crime statistics, which annually indicate high numbers of crimes that are "drug related" (66 percent in recent statistics). But this is misleading. Drug use and trade are criminalized in South Africa, and the statistics refer to incidents or arrests relating to use or trade. The link is not clearly that drug use leads to crime, but rather that drug use *is* the crime. Property-related crime in no way intimates that the properties themselves cause the crime, but somehow in drug-related crime, drugs tend to be positioned as the guilt agents. Like these crime statistics, the campaign played a game of confirmatory trickery, affirming what everyone already "knew." Standing ideas and the circulation and confirmation of set perspectives create certainty in "knowledge" that stands on shaky grounds, as could be seen in the Matrix clinic.

OPENING LINES

At the start of every Matrix meeting, the "clients" sat in a circle in the group room and introduced themselves by giving their names and the number of days they were "clean and sober." Each introduction was followed by applause from the rest of the group no matter how many "clean" days the person announced, though it was painfully obvious when someone's count, which had been steadily climbing toward recognized goals (twenty days, fifty days, sixty days . . .) and corresponding gifts (a key ring, a cup, a water-bottle . . .), suddenly dipped down to zero or single figures. At best, such a plunge indicated "lapse" or a moment of faltering in the form of a drink, a drag, a spike, a puff, or even the use of a painkiller of the "wrong" type. Or it might signal a "relapse"—a more extended period of return to what was described as "active" use. (Though the corollary "inactive use" made no sense, this framing indicated that people could never quite get away from their status as "abusers" even if use was in the distant past.) Admission was not seen as a bad thing: confession opened the space for group support and censure. Both played an important part of socializing what was hoped to be new, abstinent forms of existence.

The circle of people introducing themselves, the aim of abstinence, the tokens for periods of success, and the confessional mode are all easily recognizable as mirroring the opening of Alcoholics or Narcotics Anonymous (AA/NA) support groups anywhere in the world. Founded in America in the 1930s on the heels of prohibition, AA presents habitual substance use as—at its essence—a personal, moral failing. The AA/NA framing is that the human condition is naturally weak and requiring of spiritual guidance, and that habitual substance use results from an individual failure to accept God (Hansen 2013) and an inability to see and assess the self with accuracy (Carr 2013). Consequently, healing (or "recovery") requires connection to a "higher power," acknowledgment of personal fallibility and powerlessness; overcoming self-deception; and group communion in abstinence from all substances (except tobacco). Healing further requires facing one's wrongs and reconnecting with other people. This latter point is important because it grounds the widely assumed notion that people who use substances are external to society, not part of kin and community.

This "moral model" has a long reach—temporal and geographic. In South Africa, there are currently 350 AA groups listed online.[6] These are accompanied by other groups that are variations on the theme: Narcotics Anonymous, Sex Addicts Anonymous, Overeaters Anonymous, and Gambling Anonymous groups all have active local chapters. Other treatment centers similarly build on AA foundations, though a number of facilities are based on Islamic principles, too.

This religious orientation makes sense in the national context. South Africa is a secular state with a monotheistic heart—84 percent of people identify as Christian and a further 2 percent as Muslim (Schoeman 2017)—and so these religious overtones resonate comfortably. It is the absence of religion from treatment that sits uncomfortably for many. The extent of this was striking at a conference in Cape Town, disconcertingly entitled "More than just a junkie," about substance (ab)use in the city. The organizer assured me that the name was a purposeful attempt at raising hackles to further the conversation away from restrictive moral perspectives. Given that the hackles raised were those of the people already arguing against those same restrictive moral perspectives, this was unconvincing. At the end of the first day, a speaker presenting her work argued that in her research, "addicts" had repeatedly referred to their need for a higher power in their healing process. She therefore recommended that religious values be a required part of treatment approaches and programs. Even atheists, she argued, could not object to this, because they also believed in something, even if that something was nothing. Satisfied murmurs of assent rippled through the audience, the majority social workers based in treatment centers. The logical fallacy of the argument—as well described by Summerson Carr (2010)—is that when people are repeatedly told they need a higher power to heal in a context where confessional self-critique is lauded, this becomes a mantra that replicates and reinforces itself.

DISEASE AND BLAME

Despite the multiple resonances with the twelve-step AA model, the Matrix Programme also distances itself from twelve-step theory and practice. In particular, Matrix programmes are presented as "evidence-based"[7] and emphasize that addiction is a disease of the brain. The brain-disease framing gained traction when Alan Leshner, then the director of the U.S. National Institute on Drug Abuse (NIDA), published an opinion piece in *Nature* in which he described addiction as a "chronic, relapsing, brain disorder" (Leshner 1997, 45).

Drawing on brain imaging, the disease model explains habitual substance use in terms of neural functioning. Addiction is described as a consequence of substance use overstimulating the production of dopamine (the feel-good neurotransmitter), resulting in the body being unable to produce enough itself, therefore leading to the ongoing need to stimulate this through external (substance) means. Hereditary predisposition and personality type (also hereditary) are framed as the reasons why some people find themselves tied into compulsive drug use, while others do not.[8] Treatment center experience and data provide seemingly solid evidence of this framing in the dismal treatment success rate (where success is defined as the achievement of abstinence), with 8 percent documented in American treatment centers (Goodfellow 2008). Supporters of this "disease model" point out that this biological understanding, and the concept of compulsion, removed moral valences: the affected person is a victim of their biology, rather than guilty of a moral or spiritual failing, and therefore worthy of being treated as a patient suffering an illness.

Claiming science, asserting compassion, and supported by the next acting director of NIDA, Michael Botticelli, at a time when 85 percent drug use research was funded by NIDA (Hall, Carter, and Forlini 2015), the disease model soared to theoretical and applied dominance. It was worked into the definition of addiction presented by the highly influential American Society of Addiction Medicine (Hall, Carter, and Forlini 2015) and became widely used in health settings and treatment centers.[9]

Yes despite assertions that the disease model is distinct from the moral model, these approaches became thoroughly entangled in treatment centers (Hansen 2013; Garriott 2013)—perhaps because the disease model has limited reach. The concept of compulsion can reduce blame on the person continuing to use substances, but it does not unseat the blame for starting use. As one of the nurses in DP Marais said, not without sympathy, "I wonder why? I wonder how? Why do they start that, if, if, they know it is not good? Because everybody knows it is not good, but they still do it." In this, the shift away from judgment is incomplete. As Hammer and colleagues (2013) have pointed out, having a disease is itself not stigma free, especially if there is a potential link with behavior, even if that link is irrelevant. For example, people who develop lung cancer experience stigma even if they have never smoked (Chapple, Ziebland, and McPherson 2004). Therapeutic programs are still designed as processes of supported individual self-realization that are aimed at transforming the personhood of the individual in treatment (Zigon 2010) because ceasing use is still seen to require a combination of "motivation, commitment and tackling physical dependency" (Buchanan 2004, 118). Willpower or its lack remains central to the failure to achieve abstinence, and the character of a person using substance still has their character at stake.

Despite this conceptual confusion, the disease model has held sway. In 2014, when I was conducting most of this research, it was unquestionably the dominant model in South African academia. The same year, an editorial in the journal *Nature* claimed that "none of [the disease model explanation] is particularly controversial, at least among scientists." This assumption of unity galvanized an vocal eruption of dissenting voices. A response letter, signed by ninety-four scientists, argued that "substance abuse cannot be divorced from its social, psychological, cultural, political, legal and environmental contexts: it is not *simply* a consequence of brain malfunction" (Heim 2014, emphasis mine). The word "simply" here is important, because—in a polarized environment where theories are pitted against each other—it implies complexity. The letter also clearly stated the point that anthropologists have been making, evidently without sufficient traction in other disciplines, for over seventy years. Substance use, its effects, and modes of response cannot be divorced from context.

ANTHROPOLOGICAL INPUTS

How has the discipline of anthropology explained and explored substance use? Merrill Singer (2012) classifies historical anthropological approaches into four models. The "cultural model," initiated in the 1950s, examined the experiences and consequences of alcohol use, showing that not only the social but also the physical consequences of inebriation are culturally mediated. "Very drunk" does not necessarily equate to "hangover in the making," nor is "very drunk very often" necessarily a path to "addiction." In the 1960s and 1970s, "lifestyle model" anthropologists turned to presenting drug use in terms of the meaning ascribed to certain substances by the subcultures that used them. A focus on macro-level structures and drug use as a consequence of inequalities, dispossession, and control came to the fore with "critical medical anthropology," which gained steam from the early 1980s. The more recent "experiential model" emphasizes the lived realities and experiences of drug use and treatment within a political economic framework.[10] Experiential model work, I find, falls into two loose clusters: studies of substance use as constitutive of sociality, identity, and citizenship, as well as studies of therapeutic and health care responses as cultural processes. I outline both briefly, because both influence and situate this book and make powerful if underacknowledged claims about substance use as a social phenomenon. Work in the first "social" cluster shows that substance use is not necessarily the blade that severs relationships and makes self-serving islands out of people, but can, rather, be the stuff of belonging. Love, sharing, and deep, intimate care are part of life for people who use substances (Bourgois and Schonberg 2009).[11] Family relations may be forged through substance use (Garcia 2010; Saris 2013), and substance use can channel the movement of people through the world and foster identities (Lovell 2013). We are provided with a very different image to the specter of the addict-outcast who needs to be reconnected with society. This serves as a fundamental reminder that people who use substances retain their humanity and worth, and it stands in stark relief to comments such as, "They are going to die anyway. . . ." Work in this cluster also shows us that substance use frequently occurs in conditions of inequality and that intensifying marginalization and increased drug use go hand in hand (Brown 2010; Bourgois and Schonberg 2009; Garcia 2010; Versfeld 2012), as do racial discrimination and substance use (Goodfellow 2008). Here, the causative agents of substance use are unrealized citizenship and the ways that structural constraints suffocate the possibilities of a dignified life. Blame takes a different seat: if "they" die, it will be of neglect.

Studies of therapeutic and health care responses—the second cluster—have shown the extent to which the language and processes of treatment centers are not neutral. Rather, treatment models instill the very narratives that are then read as evidence (Carr 2010, 2013). (They say they need a higher power, so it must be true. . . .) Assumptions of inevitable relapse do the work of cementing the position of "the sick," by preempting individuals' repeated "relapses," and foreclosing possibilities of long-term healing (Campbell 2013; Garcia 2008, 2010; Schüll 2013). Furthermore, the therapeutically imagined experience of use does not necessarily reflect the actual experience of use, and treatment center workers, clients, and clients' families may all interpret evidence of success differently (Meyers 2013).

An additional area of anthropological enquiry—most notably engaged, applied work—came into being with the advent of the "harm reduction" approach. Anthropologists working alongside service providers in persuading people who use drugs to use harm reduction services (and noting when they do not) have served to point out that interventions based on ungrounded epidemiological findings are off the mark and have been advisors that shape projects to local context and the needs (Campbell and Shaw 2008; Maher 2002; Bourgois 2002; Power 2002; Moore 1993).[12] This embedded anthropological engagement has not been without difficulties or critics. The harm reduction approach of meeting people "where they are at" is presented as nonpolitical. However, the approach can frame people who use substances as predominantly of interest because of their "risk" profiles (Bourgois et al. 1997; Carroll 2011). This approach can also cast people using substances as agential neoliberal subjects, free to make choices relating to their health, while downplaying the ways in which structural constraints foster substance use and limit choices (Moore and Fraser 2006; Bourgois et al. 1997). Harm reduction can also unwittingly be implemented to the exclusion of women (Carroll 2011), and a gendered approach is generally relatively new to the field. Yet Officer P—who had likely assumed my position by virtue of the organization that had contracted me—was not wrong. The harm reduction approach is one that has resonated with me, as I turn to it in the latter parts of this book. Here I also turn to the somewhat disconcerting fact that the wealth of anthropological work and evidence to date has not swayed popular opinion toward acknowledgment of the social dynamics of drug use. Rather, it took an old set of experiments with rats.

THE PERSUASIVE POWER OF RATS

In the late 1970s and early 1980s, Bruce Alexander led an experiment with rats examining the impact of social environment and isolation on substance use (Alexander et al. 1981). The experiment, affectionately called "Rat Park" by the researchers, was designed to counter prior studies that had shown that rats held in experimental conditions with access to addictive substances would imbibe large amounts, which was read as proof of the biological basis of addiction. In the study conducted by Alexander and colleagues, newly weaned rats were divided into two groups. Rats in one group were divided up and housed in isolation. Rats in the other group were housed in a colony with place to play, socialize, and mate. After a period, half the rats were swapped so that those who had been isolated could socialize and vice versa. Then both groups were given unlimited access to water and morphine hydrochloride. The key finding—that rats in colonies imbibed markedly less morphine than their isolated counterparts, no matter how they had started out—was described as "large and robust" (Alexander et al. 1981, 574) by the study authors. Yet, unlike prior studies, the finding was not broadly extrapolated to people by others in the field. Then, in 2010, Alexander published a book in which he repackaged the argument about habitual substance use as a product of social disconnection—bolstered with historical and anthropological records (Alexander 2010). The concept gained traction. A 2013 evocative long-form comic strip by Stuart McMillen, 2015 Ted Talk by the journalist John Hari (currently standing at over 16 million views), and a documentary on the experiment produced in 2019 turned the Rat Park experiment into a kind of "popular parable" (to use Alexander's phrase)[13] that explained why people use substances.

In this form, the "social model" has risen to prominence and been sharpened into a conceptual weapon that is used to disprove the disease model. Both the social and disease models, however, risk self-destruction when they are wielded in all-encompassing ways. Context matters, but so do the physical realities such as the extreme discomfort of withdrawal from opioids and the attraction of the sensation of use (or of the gentle absence of sensation) that opioids can lead to. Habitual substance use—individual and group—is a messy mix of physiological responses to substance, social conditions, dispossession, and cultural patterns and responses. This recognition, however, makes for no clear narrative and requires stepping away from the attractive comfort of a "single story" (Adichie 2009; Mkhwanazi 2016). (If "they" die, who is to blame? Well . . . everyone.) In some cases, the moral, disease, and social models are used together in contradictory ways, not so much to acknowledge complexity, but rather because each serves a different need. The result, as South African drug policy shows, can be a hot mess.

SOUTH AFRICA'S POLICY POSITION ON DRUG USE

South Africa's drug policy is periodically reviewed and set out in National Drug Master Plans (NDMPs), with the most recent, fourth version, released in 2020.[14] At the time of most of the ethnographic research undertaken for this book, the third NDMP (released in 2013) was in play. A 167-page document, it runs the gamut of basic errors: conceptual inconsistencies are adorned by grammar and typological errors, inviting dismissal from serious academic engagement. (Where is one to start with a productive critique?) Nevertheless, the third NDMP was the key reference document that set out the country's position on substance use, and it was frequently referred to in official discussions. It therefore mattered that in it, people who used drugs were firmly located as to blame for their own use (Howell and Couzyn 2015; Pienaar and Savic 2015). It was a concern that calls for evidence-based responses coexisting with a dearth of evidence available about the scope, scale, or dynamics of drug use. The document rested, rather, on well-worn hyperbole, making—for example—unsubstantiated claims of drug (ab)use continuing to "ravage families, communities and society" (Department of Social Development, Central Drug Authority 2013, 2). This was the first time harm reduction appeared in national policy, but it did so in a contorted form.

While concerns about health and the spread of HIV underwrote the acceptance of the harm reduction approach to drug use in the rest of the world, South Africa wielded health in a different way in drug policy. The first NDMP, published in 1999, aimed to address "health risks and other damages associated with drug misuse, including the spread of communicable diseases, related injuries and premature death" (1999). The second National Drug Master Plan (2006–2011) added "special areas of concern," including "substance abuse among people of childbearing age . . . teenage pregnancy, fetal alcohol syndrome, multidrug resistance and sexually transmitted infections, including HIV and AIDS" (2006, 16). The third National Drug Master Plan (2013–2017) spread the net wider, to include early death, the effects on people experiencing violent crime, "accidents and deaths of innocent drivers," the "psychological impacts" on family members, and "social ills faced by communities under siege" (2013, 2). Each expanded list of health and wellness concerns served to justify the growing emphasis on the argument that healthy communities require that substance use be eliminated. This was coupled with a corresponding increasing focus on punishment, rehabilitation, and contraction of individual rights across these first three policy documents.

Given this trajectory, it is hardly surprising that when, in 2013, harm reduction was included as an ideal, in the NDMP, it appeared in a "localized" form, defined as "limiting or ameliorating the damage caused to individuals or communities who have already succumbed to the temptation of substance abuse." Passing reference to the more common understanding of harm reduction as reducing the negative impact of drug use is maintained, but people who use drugs are no longer the focus of care.[15] This adaptation is justified by noted concerns that, as internationally defined, "harm reduction practices appear to condone drug use," something framed as intolerable given that drug use is "criminalized by the state" and in "medical terms the action taken should be seen to be preventative" (2013, 68). The use of the term "harm reduction" indicates a recognition of the importance of the concept, but the reassignment of meaning shows a fundamental rejection of the values it implies. If national policy cannot see harm reduction as relevant to health or applicable to "our people," it is hardly surprising that law enforcement officers do not.

How is it that a country that has produced one of the most progressive constitutions in the world can produce drug policy that is incoherent and dismissive of human rights? The 1996 South African Constitution demonstrates a deep regard for the value of each individual, guaranteeing the right to equality, dignity, life, and access to health care services. The Constitution provides for all people to have the right to freedom from discrimination based on a litany of stated criteria.[16] The uncomfortable fact at play here is that the rights enshrined in the Constitution do not enjoy the popular support of the people[17] or, evidently, the policy makers. But perhaps the more important issue is that the Constitution is at odds with international legislative frameworks, which legitimates a conflicting policy approach.

South Africa is signatory to—among others—the UNODC 1961 Single Convention on Narcotic Drugs and the Convention Against Illicit Traffic in Narcotic Drugs and Psychotropic Substances, 1988. These two frameworks and the national laws that flow from them criminalize drug use and trade, and make abstinence not just the ideal but the only way to be a law-abiding citizen. Stigma and discrimination find fertile ground. As one of the delegates suggested at a drug policy meeting in South Africa in 2017, poor treatment of people who use drugs by health care providers is, internationally, perhaps one of the last remaining bastions of accepted medical disregard for the dignity and autonomy of patients.

The impetus provided by international drug laws also pulls in opposite directions to the approaches of various international health institutions. The various UN bodies, the WHO, and—for TB—the StopTB Partnership have all shifted toward a harm reduction approach in the past decade, emphasizing the need to focus on the health of citizens, no matter what their drug use patterns. The Global Fund, which provides the greatest health funding to lower- and middle-income countries, both funds harm reduction and—in recent calls—emphasizes the need for funding proposals to include harm reduction interventions. Governments and health ministries are accountable to these institutions, not least because acting in accordance with guidelines and protocols is a funding requirement.

The way these tensions are managed at a national level depends on dominant local perspectives and mandates. In South Africa, drug policy is the ambit of the Central Drug Authority, an organization housed within the Department of Social Development but made up of representatives of twenty-one government departments, including the Departments of Health, Correctional Services, Justice and Constitutional Development and International Relations and Co-operation, and 13 independent experts. Each of these institutions comes to the policy development table with different mandates, priorities, and perspectives (Stein and Manyedi 2016). The National Department of Health is responsible for managing medical emergencies, medical complications, detoxification, and comorbidities relating to drug use. This demands a very different set of priorities to those of law enforcement agencies (including the South African Police Service and the Departments of Correctional Services and of Justice), which are obligated to follow international legal frameworks in aiming for a "South Africa free of substance abuse." Individuals representing these institutions are also products of the common (mis)conceptions of how and why people use substances. Shifting toward a less punitive approach requires agreement from a multitude of parties, many of whom have no obligation to be informed about what the evidence really is. The criminalization of drug use does not always result in punitive law enforcement processes; in some countries, police support needle and syringe programs, or even safe injecting rooms—Malaysia and the United Kingdom provide good respective examples (Monaghan and Bewley-Taylor 2013). As others have illustrated, the bland presentation of policy belies the ways in which it is not neutral, but rather made to fit and bolster existing agendas (Tate 2015; Fassin 2007). But in South African drug policy development, we see how practicalities, moralities, and mandates collide.

DISSONANCE AT THE HIGHEST LEVELS

Perhaps the greatest demonstration of dissonance and disagreement within South African leadership about the direction drug policy should take was its recently subterfuge at the highest levels. In 2016, the UN General Assembly held its first general meeting with a focus on drugs. In preparation for this meeting, African Union countries gathered and developed a Common Position Paper. This called for a less punitive, more rights-focused continental approach to drugs. The deputy minister of the South African Department of Social Development took a leadership role in developing the paper and was mandated to make the official presentation of this new position at an United Nations General Assembly (UNGASS) premeeting in Vienna. However, the day before the presentation, the deputy minister found that her name had quietly been removed from the speakers list, replaced by the South African ambassador to Austria, presenting an alternative document, called the "African Group Position Paper." This latter document did not come from the African Union, but rather from a small group of African countries that had been concerned about the direction of the

African Union position. Representatives from these countries had quietly met and drafted a more conservative alternative. The ambassador to Vienna was also South Africa's representative on the Atomic Energy Board, and since the Atomic Energy Board happened to be in the same building as the Commission on Narcotic Drugs, he doubled up and represented South African on the Commission, too. What ensued was a back and forth, with the deputy minister placing her name back on the speakers list, to have it removed again. In the end she spoke, but as a representative of the African Union, not South Africa. Subsequently, the South African ambassador to Austria submitted the more conservative Group Position Paper as the official position of the African Union. The sleight of hand, in which domestic conservatism trumped international responsibility, was only uncovered later.

The tug of war between drug policy reformers and conservatives has played out again in the development and release of the most recent (fourth) version of the NDMP. In the drug policy advocacy world, there was appreciation of the fact that people who use drugs had been consulted in the development of this new NDMP, and there was a tangible hope that the document would set out a brave new landscape. However, as the old policy document passed its sell-by date, the new policy document continued through multiple rounds of comments and inputs and was somehow never finalized. Eventually, the nineteenth incarnation was passed by parliament in November 2019, but its public release took another eight months. While the final document is a notable departure from the past in that it recognizes the social basis of drug use and (re)defines harm reduction for South Africa to align with a WHO definition, indicating that "harm reduction interventions are evidence-based public health principles to support people who use drugs," it has also, according to people who saw previous versions, been stripped of all the measures that would have cemented a less punitive approach and had previously been included.

SUBSTANCE USE IN TB POLICY

Prior to 1994, South African TB response efforts had largely been through ad hoc efforts of containment within the "African" community (Churchyard et al. 2014; Packard 1989). While the new government sought to integrate and improve a fractured primary health care system that could provide equally for all the population, TB rates started to surge as the HIV epidemic started to take hold. In 1996, the government declared TB a national emergency and set up the first National Tuberculosis Control Programme (Republic of South Africa 2004).

Early national TB guidelines drew on the first set of guidelines issued in 1993 by the WHO. Substance use is absent from these early guidelines, first appearing in the guidelines for managing drug-resistant TB issued in 2011 and updated in 2013. (These are henceforth referred to as "the South African Guidelines.") The

WHO "Guidelines for Programmatic Management of Drug-Resistant Tuberculosis" of 2006 (henceforth the "WHO Guidelines") serve as a blueprint for
the South African guidelines. In relation to substance use, however, the South
African guidelines have minor (but telling) alterations.

The WHO Guidelines (2006) read:

> Patients with substance dependence disorders should be offered treatment for
> their addiction. Complete abstinence from alcohol or other substances should
> be strongly encouraged, although active consumption is not a contraindication
> for anti-TB treatment. If the treatment is repeatedly interrupted because of the
> patient's dependence, therapy should be suspended until successful treatment or
> measures to ensure adherence have been established. (World Health Organi-
> zation 2006, 65)

The South African Guidelines (2013) read:

> Substance Dependency Patients who abuse alcohol and drugs should be started
> on a rehabilitation programme and if necessary adjuvant therapy given. Although
> complete abstinence from alcohol or drugs should be strongly encouraged, treat-
> ment is not contraindicated in people who abuse alcohol or drugs. If the treatment
> is repeatedly interrupted due to the patient's addiction, then it should be sus-
> pended until successful rehabilitation or other measures to ensure adherence are
> established. (Republic of South Africa 2013, 79)

The WHO Guidelines refer to "substance dependence disorders" and suggest
the offer of "treatment for addiction," drawing on the language of the *DSM-IV*,[18]
which presents the official view of the disease model of substance use. The word
"abuse"—a term impossible to uncouple from moral censure—does not appear
in the WHO Guidelines at all but appears twice in this short section of the South
African Guidelines and a further nine times in the South African guidelines
overall, always in relation to drugs.

The suggestion in the WHO Guidelines of the "offer" of treatment indicates
that the person using substances is in control of their choice about whether to
start treatment or not. The South African Guidelines take a notably less gentle
approach, indicating that "people should be started on a rehabilitation programme" or given "adjuvant therapy" (the latter would, for example, be medication that makes the patient extremely sick if they use alcohol). "Offer" is
turned into requirement, and the will of the patient recedes from view.

The WHO Guidelines indicate that if dependence results in TB treatment interruption (this itself is an assumption we will deal with later), then TB medication
should be stopped until "successful treatment [for the substance use]" or "other
measures to ensure adherence are established." While "successful treatment" could

be the cessation of substance use, it could also be opioid substitution therapy. The South African Guidelines refer to "successful rehabilitation," with the term "rehabilitation" implying that the substance-using person needs to return to an ideal state of abstinence. Elsewhere in the South African Guidelines, it is similarly stated, under the heading "social support," that "patients who are substance abusers must be started on rehabilitation programmes with intensive counselling as [TB] treatment compliance tends to be poor in this group of patients" (2013, 94).

As the international guidelines are adapted to national preference, they have been shaped to align with local conceptions of what is good and proper—and therefore deserving of care.[19] In doing so, the South African Guidelines set up a conundrum: TB treatment facilities are required to send people who use substances to substance use treatment facilities, but these facilities will not (and cannot) treat patients with infectious TB due to fears of infection spread, especially if the infected person is not seeking to attain abstinence. Morality trumps practicality (never mind rights), and the guidelines are rendered impossible to follow.

CONCLUSION

Local evidence about the extent and dynamics of substance use has, historically, been lacking. Opinions and perspectives on substance use have tended to be based on moral perspectives, making them extremely sticky and hard to shift. This trend is not unique to South Africa, nor is as extreme as it might be. In the Philippines, for example, President Duterte has led a killing spree of people who use drugs (Simangan 2018). In a number of other East and Southeast Asian countries, people who use drugs can be held in compulsory detention centers merely on the suspicion of drug use. However, the realities of the effects of South African policy positions are lived daily by people who use drugs as they struggle to access health care, find themselves stigmatized and poorly treated when they do access care (Scheibe, Shelly, and Versfeld 2020), and are repeatedly harassed, sometimes physically abused, and arrested by police. Most of these realities do not enter into this book, which examines the more subtle effects of these policy positions, but they should be kept in mind as a backdrop to the events and situations described here.

This has set up a practical dilemma in the provision of TB treatment for people who use substances. What should happen with TB patients who are using substances if they cannot receive TB treatment until they have gone through substance use treatment (and achieved abstinence) and they cannot receive substance use treatment if they are infectious with TB? This dilemma only stands as long as abstinence is regarded as necessary for TB treatment, something that the TB policy correctly indicates is not a physiological requirement. It is also, I suggest, a dilemma that has been created by another problematic assumption inherent in both the old WHO treatment guidelines and the current South African policy document. This is that it is substance use per se that dislodges the chances of successful TB treatment. I go on to illustrate in subsequent chapters that although the link between TB, treatment default, and substance use is clear, there has not been enough attention to the forces that meld these links. There has been too little questioning of how the public health care system (and those who work within it) has set up the dynamics in which patients avoid the health care system, interrupt treatment, and cycle in and out of care in relation to substance use–TB co-constitution.

3 · CO-CONSTITUTIONS
Makers and Maskers

THE NARRATIVES THAT MATTER

Dr N,[1] the doctor who oversees the women's ward, is busy on her ward round when she notices Lucinda, bone-thin and newly arrived, come in from outside and get into bed. "Have we met before?" Dr N asks, unsure of whether this is Lucinda's first admission to DP Marais. "Um-mmm," says Lucinda, in a mutter of the negative. "Welcome!" says Dr N.

A few minutes later, having completed her conversation with another patient, Dr N goes to Lucinda's bed, where she encloses them both (and me) with a curtain, and requests permission for my presence while they chat. Lucinda acquiesces, but does not acknowledge me further in any way.

"You need to tell me nicely what's going on,"[2] Dr N says, and asks which hospital sent Lucinda to DP Marais. Lucinda names a local tertiary hospital, her tone is reticent. "Why did you go there?" Dr N asks. "The TB came back," Lucinda replies, simply. "It looks like you kept defaulting [treatment]," says Dr N as she pages through Lucinda's file. She comments that Lucinda started treatment in 2013, but did not finish. "What's stopping you finishing?" she queries. Lucinda, sounding frustrated, says, "I stay outside. I sleep outside. . . ."

"Do you stay alone, or with others?" Dr N asks. "On my own," says Lucinda. "That must be scary," Dr N commiserates. Lucinda says it is. She is lying down, closing her eyes some of the time.

Dr N asks if Lucinda has ever been tested for HIV. "I am HIV," Lucinda says, and through leaving out the word "positive" she merges her identity with the illness in a way I have not heard before. Dr N asks Lucinda where and when she found this out. She says in 2004, then, angry she says, "You speak so loudly!" Dr N says not to worry, the people in the beds next to her only speak isiXhosa.

"Are you still taking [antiretroviral therapy]?" Dr N asks. She is not. "Why not?" "Because I sleep outside, what must I do with them?" Lucinda's annoyance is clear. Dr N asks her where she will go when she leaves here, the hospital. Lucinda says that she will go and stay with her mother.

"Why?" Dr N asks, was she not staying with her mother before? "No reason," says Lucinda. Dr N presses her; there must be a reason. "No reason," Lucinda repeats, stoic in her refusal to get drawn into a conversation. Dr N asks her why she will go back to her mother now. She does not want to be alone.

Dr N asks her when her TB tablets started. "Monday." When did she get sick, and what were her symptoms? Dr N wants to know. "TB symptoms," says Lucinda, not very helpfully. Dr N asks what those were. "Coughing, shortness of breath. . . ." Lucinda trails off. "Weight loss?" prompts Dr N. "Hmmm," affirms Lucinda. "Runny tummy?" Dr N prompts again. "Every now and again. . . ."

Dr N notes that Lucinda was also in a local day hospital for about ten days. Dr N asks her about blood tests, "Did they tell you there is a germ in your blood?" Lucinda replies in the negative, "No, they didn't tell me anything."

"Does your mother know you are here?" Dr N asks. "No, man, can you do me a favor?" Lucinda asks, with the first hint of enthusiasm for the conversation. She says her mother knew she was in the local day hospital, but doesn't know she is here. She asks Dr N to please call her, giving the number. It is a different number to the one in the file, which causes some confusion. Dr N says that her files indicate that in a previous TB episode treatment she had completed the course and she asks about any other medical problems. Lucinda "hmphs" a negative.

"Do you have any questions?" Dr N wants to know. Another "hmph" in the negative. Dr N continues to press on. "How long have you been living on the street?" she asks. "Two or three years," replies Lucinda. Dr N asks if Lucinda is married. She is not.

"Do you have children?" Dr N does not give up. "One. A boy," says Lucinda "Where does he live?" asks Dr N. "In a house," replies Lucinda, both evading the question and implying that he is better off than he would be if he was with her, on the street. "But in which area?" Dr N presses. Lucinda names an area close to the last hospital she attended.

Dr N keeps on seeking a place of connection, "Does he go to school?" He does. "Is he clever?" Thwarting Dr N's effort at finding a place of easier communication, Lucinda replies, "Stupid." Dr N utters a sound of surprise and Lucinda, softening a bit, says, "Oh, he's okay. . . ."

Changing tack, Dr N asks Lucinda if she smokes. "Two to three per day," says Lucinda. Dr N clarifies, "How many cigarettes do you smoke?" The number jumps up to 15. The "two to three" was clearly about something else. "Tik, dagga, mandrax . . . ?" Dr N probes in a half formed question of common local drugs. "Heroin," says Lucinda. Dr N asks her when last she smoked. "Two weeks ago."

"Does your mom know?" Dr N asks. She does. "Is she happy?" queries Dr N. "No, she is not happy," says Lucinda, noticeably annoyed again. "Do you have withdrawals?" asks Dr N. "Yes!" Lucinda affirms. "Tell me about them. . . ." Dr N requests, but Lucinda is done with all these questions. "Doctor, I'm not going to talk anymore." And when Dr N asks, "Are you tired?" there is no reply. "We're going to talk lots more about this in the future," says Dr N. (Field notes, DP Marais TB Hospital, August 2014)

Lucinda's intake interview stayed with me. It was a halting, verbal dance of an interaction (step, step, misstep, try a different approach and direction) that demonstrates so much about the complexity of navigating conversations about health and substance use in the medical setting. It shows how the patient and the doctor were not quite adversaries, but neither, in the context of substance use, were they collaborators. Rather, they were working out how to place each other, what could be said, and what—in the context of substance use—was best left unsaid. But there was something else going on, too. Lucinda's unveiled frustration when asked why, this time, she was defaulting on her TB treatment ("I stay outside. I sleep outside . . .") and why she was not consistently on her ART ("Because I sleep outside, what must I do with them?") suggested that her personal explanation for her poor health lay, ultimately, in her living conditions. Over the years of talking with people with TB, I have consistently found that while most (though certainly not all) have known that a pathogen is a necessary condition for their illness, many have explained the cause of their illness as individual life conditions, whether these are work situations, living arrangements (or lack of them), care relations, familial structures, or substance use. The pathogen takes a back seat in the conversation. How else is someone to understand and explain that TB has taken root in and taken over their body, while others around them, living much the same lives, have been spared?

This is a chapter about how the constitution of health and illness is understood and, consequently, what the best course of action is seen to be. It is about what is said and what is left unsaid. It is also about what is made and what is hidden when TB and substance use come together. Through exploring this particular co-constitution, I examine how the ways that health forces interact in the development of poor health are understood by health care providers and people affected. As I do this, I build a critique of syndemic theory, which is increasingly being used to illustrate, explore, and explain the ways that diseases and health conditions come together under conditions of inequality. I show how current framings of syndemic theory can encourage a pathologization of life patterns and inherently privilege biological interactions as if these, ultimately, define health states. I further foreground an area that has been underexplored in the syndemics literature—the ways in which co-constituting health forces are powerful in their capacities to redirect bodily experiences (for people affected) and readings of illness (for health care providers), obfuscating understandings of why poor health is happening.

BABALWA: A LIFE OF GATHERING "RISK FACTORS"

Babalwa arrived in the hospital with a referral letter that described a complex litany of "medical" issues, including HIV (and not on treatment), a "productive" cough and other constitutional symptoms of TB, dysentery, chronic headaches, wasting, and high and swinging fevers. At the bottom, it included a "social" reason for admission to DP Marais: history nonadherence. And over the page another note: "Patient at high risk of defaulting, needs placement at DP Marais. . . ."

Babalwa remained in the hospital for almost six months, until the end of her treatment for drug-sensitive TB. During this period, she religiously attended the substance (ab)use awareness sessions in the hospital, although it was clear that as a Xhosa first language speaker, she frequently could not follow the discussions, which were held in English and Afrikaans. In one meeting, the participants, who were seated in a circle, would each answer a question about their lives. Each time it was Babalwa's turn to answer, the flow of answers would come to a halt. Whatever the question was, she would sit forward nervously, rub her hands up and down her thighs, and hesitantly say the same thing: "I want to leave the bad things I was doing. I want to be a mother and father to my children because I don't have any family. . . ." Wendy, the substance (ab)use coordinator,[3] would repeat the question (though louder). Babalwa's reply was less an answer and more a plea to herself: "I want to leave the bad things I was doing, I want to be a mother and father to my children because I don't have any family. . . ." She did not rail at the cruelty of apartheid, poverty, failed leadership in the face of HIV, and the general unkindness of the world. Rather, as was the culture of the group sessions, her guilt-stricken expression of individual accountability was repeated like a mantra, and the other group members giggled and rolled their eyes, further ostracizing her. Perhaps, had they known her life story, some empathy would have pierced the room and someone would have taken her hand and said, "This is not your fault," for her life is demonstrative of the rough road of life in poverty in South Africa and how her poor health was all but forewritten (Ross 2010).

Babalwa was born in the late 1970s in the Transkei, an area that is now the Eastern Cape designated a "homeland" (or "Bantustans") by the apartheid government.[4] Homelands were pockets of largely rural land to which Black South Africans were forcibly moved during apartheid. Ten specific areas were designated for particular (apartheid-defined, anthropologist-described) ethnic groups around the country. Homelands were provided with nominal independence, but this was only recognized by South Africa. In reality, they were completely reliant on the South African economy and run by leaders functioning—at least to some extent—at the behest of the apartheid government. The rolling hills and lush coastline of the Transkei could not support the sudden influx of people, and the land—overgrazed and underserviced—quickly became degraded, infertile, and riven by "dongas" (deep, eroded gullies). Most families in the areas survived on wage remittances of migrant family members working in "White South Africa" (the official phrase for the country excluding the homelands). Education was limited, and the school curriculum was designed for limiting life opportunities to labor. Formal health services were almost nonexistent. The social fabric of these areas was frayed by poverty and land pressure and stripped by migrant labor and the consequences of overarching oppression and dispossession.

Aged three, Babalwa was struck by her first major life tragedy; she was orphaned when both her parents were accused of witchcraft and murdered. From then on until her late teens, she was raised by her grandmother and together they eked a rough, rural survival. Then, when she was in her late teens, her grandmother died. Bereft and without family that would support her (though she did have an uncle in the area), Babalwa went to seek a living and a life in Cape Town. On arrival in the city, she stayed with a friend in one of the many townships distant from the city center, but work proved elusive. Her friend, pragmatic and schooled in city survival, informed her that she had better find a boyfriend, someone who could, at least, buy her toiletries. This she did and not long after she became pregnant and gave birth to a son. The child's father provided life's essentials and a raft of trouble. After some violent, crime-related events, Babalwa fled back to the Eastern Cape with her child, fearing for their lives. But life there proved no more sustainable than it had been when she had last left and, desperate, she returned to a different part of Cape Town. This time, she found factory work and struck up a new relationship. Approximately five years after her first child was born, she became pregnant again. The pregnancy rocked the relationship—her partner did not want her to keep the child. He gave her R500 ($33)[5] and told her to have a termination. Babalwa did not share his plans ("It is my blood!" she explained) and so she bought food with the money instead. Then, in order to hide her swelling belly, she left her employment and went back to the Eastern Cape. She returned to Cape Town late in her pregnancy, when there was no hiding her state and a termination was no longer a possibility. Her partner, furious, refused to support her and the relationship ended. Deeply unhappy, she started to drink and continued to drink heavily through the rest of pregnancy. By this time, Babalwa had acquired HIV.[6] However, she was on antiretrovirals (ARVs) at the time of the birth, and though her baby girl was breach—which Babalwa blamed on the alcohol—she was born HIV negative.[7]

After the birth, Babalwa and her children lived in a shack in one of the populous townships of the city. She tried to survive by paying for rent and food with the pitiful money she received from government-provided child support grants.[8] At approximately $30 per month, this did not stretch to food for herself. Hunger and ART are uncomfortable partners and so she stopped her medication and staved off the worst of the hunger pangs by drinking water. In July 2013, in the depths of the wet Cape Town winter with a two-month-old baby, Babalwa found out that she had TB. In August, her own food ran out completely, her breast milk dried up, and her baby started to starve, too. In September, it occurred to Babalwa that she was dying, and so she called her uncle in the Eastern Cape to tell him. In describing her own potential death to me, she used the word "*ukufa*," the isiXhosa word used to describe a harsh death, often used for an animal rather than a person. It was a word that encapsulated the process of dying without dignity. Toward the end of September, a neighbor called an ambulance that took her to one of the largest specialist public hospitals in the city. Her baby, diarrhetic and vomiting, was taken to a specialist children's hospital. Babalwa was then transported to DP Marais, with a diagnosis of disseminated TB. Her children were both taken into state custody and put into foster care.

Babalwa's life history, as she narrated it, shows us how, in struggle and dispossession, health conditions are brought together, interweave, co-impact, and synergistically build on each other. Her story echoes that of Juan Garcia, the protagonist of a 1992 article by Merrill Singer and colleagues. Juan Garcia was a Puerto Rican immigrant in the United States who died "with a bottle in his hand and booze in his belly" (1992, 78). The authors demonstrate that the life, alcohol consumption, and death of Juan Garcia was situated in a long history of colonial oppression, dispossession from land and work, and dissociation from forms of masculinity (in both Puerto Rico and America) that did not involve drinking. Through this they illustrate that a "drinking problem" at the individual level must be understood in political-economic and historical context. Furthering this argument, Jonathan Seeberg (2013b) explores how, in India, alcohol use and TB come together in conditions of marginalization through tracing the life and death of a man called Shankar. Poor, desperate, and unable to balance work and TB treatment requirements, Shankar uses alcohol while ill despite the understanding that this will undermine his chances of healing. Seeberg shows how alcohol use and an apparent apathy to looming death are situated in the constant struggles and humiliations faced in trying to forge life and seek treatment. TB is a "bodily expression of social realities" (Seeberg 2013a, 208).

It is impossible to understand how Babalwa came to be sick almost to death unless we take into account the multiple difficulties and trials she endured as a marginalized, poor, orphaned, Black woman, born into apartheid South Africa and living without a supportive family network. We need to acknowledge how sex was one of the few resources she had at her disposal in context where HIV was endemic, largely due to a failed government response. We need to consider the ways in which TB bacilli congest in the cramped homes; how they flourish in work environments where bodies are weakened by intense exertion, airflow is limited, and dust coats workers' lungs; and how they are shared in transport methods used by marginalized people. We cannot ignore the hunger that impacted Babawa's desire to take the medication she needed to control the HIV infection in her body. And we need to note that by her own description, her illness was a consequence of hunger, stress, desperation, depression, and the balm she sought in alcohol. Hers was a life of gathering "risk factors." Yet almost none of this was in Babalwa's folder, fat as it was with "medical" information, and in the substance (ab)use treatment room, she explained her own illness in the expected narrative of self-accountability, in terms of the "bad things" she was doing.

"TREATING TB IS NOT SO STRAIGHTFORWARD . . . IT CONFUSES US ENDLESSLY"

In Cape Town in 2014, TB diagnosis was generally happening through sputum samples, which were sent to laboratories for testing. This included the quicker method examining a smear of the sputum sample under the microscope for visible bacilli to the slower, but more reliable, method of growing cultures on sputum samples. X-rays also provide a diagnostic possibility, but they were not a first diagnostic point of call as they were only available in larger hospitals, not the public health care clinics where most diagnosis was happening. Given that South Africa was also an early adopter of GeneXpert technology in the public sector, diagnosis sometimes also included genetic sequencing, especially when confirmation of TB illness was required that was not forthcoming through smear of culture processes, or if drug resistance was suspected.

None of these methods is perfect. Smears, examined under the microscope, miss positive diagnoses too often. Though more accurate, cultures take weeks to grow and may still miss present, active TB. GeneXpert results are fast and accurate (and can detect variations of drug resistance) but may provide a false-positive test result if the person being tested has recently been treated for and cured of a TB infection.[9] (A case of a person not being a "case.")[10] X-rays have historically depended on the skill of the health practitioner interpreting them and—even for the skilled practitioner—distinguishing the damage caused by TB from that of other forms of lung disease, or lung cancer, can be difficult, if not impossible.[11] On top of this all, while pulmonary TB is the most common, it is by no means the only form of TB; TB can present or hide in any organ, with symptoms that vary depending on where it manifests. This "extrapulmonary" TB is most common in immune-compromised individuals and often extremely difficult to diagnose.

Given how common TB is in resource-poor settings, it is often the fallback diagnosis when people have enough of the main symptoms (coughing, night sweats, shortness of breath, weight loss, and fever), and other explanations for these symptoms are not immediately apparent.[12] This meant that one of the first questions the hospital doctors asked themselves on the arrival of a new patient with a symptomatic diagnosis, especially when symptoms were not improving as expected with medication, was, "Does this person really have TB?" or, more accurately, "Is the likelihood that this person has TB sufficient that they should suffer the (toxic) treatment?" Once this was ascertained, if patients still were not getting better, they would be included in the weekly specialist's rounds and the question would become, "What else is going on here?"

Once a week, an infectious diseases specialist would spend a morning at the DP Marais hospital. During my research, this was Dr A. Together, he and the DP Marais doctors would walk the hospital, stopping at the beds of each patient where there were concerns about changes (or lack of them) in their health status and when biomedical treatment decisions were not obvious. These rounds involved talking, touching, tapping, and listening not just to what the patients were saying but also to the sounds of their bodies in an effort to read (or hear) the actual nature of the illness.[13] They involved the eyes, attention, and conversation of up to five doctors at one time. Sometimes they could take up to half an hour.

Felicity had first come to DP Marais with TB meningitis—a swelling of the meninges of the brain due to TB infection that can cause confusion. Her extreme poor health meant that she was set to stay in the hospital for some months. She was timid and gaunt, the form of her bones visibly pressing through her skin. And though she attended the occupational therapy sessions (when many women avoided them), she spoke little and kept her gaze cast downward. Despite this, I immediately noticed that her eyes flickered in a way I had come to know might indicate tik withdrawal. I had also learned, however, not to jump to conclusions—I had made the assumption of drug use before and been wrong. But then I heard rumors that she was dancing in the rain after her husband had come to visit. The gossip, brought into my office by another female patient, was that her moments of euphoria were brought in by her husband in the small, twisted pieces of plastic that carried tik.

A few weeks later, Felicity went home on a visit and did not reappear after the weekend as per the hospital plan (though perhaps not hers). Months later, she made an involuntary return, which I recorded in my notes:

Felicity is now back. I first heard it from Soraya, who described her as "messed up." One of the doctors was less subtle. "F***ed" was the description given, under a cupped hand as if whispering in my ear. I saw her last week, when I was walking past the women's acute ward; it has large windows, anyone can see the patients from the passage. She was tucked into a chair, arms in an awkward position. "Felicity!" I greeted, through the door. She indicated "yes" with her eyes and a slight tilt of her head. She is barely able to move, unable to talk and barely mobile—paralyzed down the right side of her body.

Felicity was propped up but slumped skew in a chair next to her bed when the cavalcade of doctors arrived in the ward. Her head wobbled, and as always, she wore a pink and purple crocheted hat. It was tipped to the side on her head, giving an additional air of things being off-kilter. As the group of doctors shifted toward her bed, she shyly wiped the crumbs of the sandwich she was struggling to eat from her cheeks with a twisted hand. Felicity sat quietly while her diagnosis, treatment, and prognosis were discussed. A recent lumber puncture had indicated that TB meningitis was not responding to the medication and it had also shown that she had latent syphilis. What was not clear was whether she had neurosyphilis, which usually appears ten to twenty years after first infection in untreated cases and can be accelerated by HIV infection. With an uncertain diagnosis, it was unclear whether she should be subjected to a ten-day course of hard-on-the-body penicillin, which might not be needed. The decision about her treatment was made, as it frequently was, by bringing it back to personal reflection. "If it was you, would you want ten days of penicillin if [your illness] was potentially treatable?" asked Dr A and, answering himself, "I think I would." Felicity was medicated for neurosyphilis, and slowly, over months, her infections came under control enough for her to be taken home into the care of her husband, something that happened after a number of meetings with the hospital medical and social staff.[14]

Medical nosology—the classification of diseases—requires that a disease is sufficiently distinct from others as to fit only into one classificatory location. This is key for how diseases are understood epistemologically and is also the basis of treatment. Medication is designed to target specific pathogens, and treatment tends to require the narrowing down of causal options of symptoms. For infectious diseases, it requires the isolation of distinct pathogens that can be pharmacologically targeted. When this is not fully apparent, best guesses serve to both increase and decrease the risks of harm being done. ("If it was you, would you want ten days of penicillin if [your illness] was potentially treatable?")

In the face of immediate and pressing medical response requirements, such as treating or not treating a patient for neurosyphilis, the role of substance use in causing or influencing disease infection and progression tended not to be regarded as being of pressing importance in the hospital, and often it slipped from view altogether. I, however, found that the questions I had about Felicity's health pressed past those discussed on the doctors' rounds. How, I wondered, had her tik use affected her illness, if at all? Had it impacted her immune system in a way that made a difference to her health outcomes? What was behind her "absconding" from the hospital? Would she, aged twenty-eight, have been sitting in a hospital chair (where she had been put by staff and would not leave until she had been taken out again) shyly wiping the crumbs off her mouth to face the group of doctors who were unsure of how and why she was not getting better? And then there were the broader questions: What was life that tik use was a refuge worthy of seeking so that she stopped taking her TB medication? What were all the threads that conspired and knotted to make her ill, and what would be needed to smooth out the knots enough for some semblance of health to be attained again?

These questions scratched at me, leaving me uncomfortable, and so I did what I had done many times before during fieldwork. I put the kettle on and settled in for a cup of coffee with Dr L, who I knew would answer me directly.

The influences and effects of substance use, he said, were often hard to determine; trying to determine whether or how it was constitutive of poor health was a game of suppositions. In contrast, focusing on isolating and treating a disease in the body was where they as a public health facility had agency. Regarding drug use as part of the background context, or a "complicating factor" in treatment and focusing on the "medical," meant that the doctors could employ the arsenal at their immediate disposal. This focus was a refuge from the fact that they were largely powerless in the face of the broader societal problems of poverty, unemployment, clinic treatment, malnutrition, and strained home or family relations, even as these materialized in substance dependence. Though the hospital staff could (and did) seek to keep some of the worst ravages of poverty at bay for individual patients through seeking to ensure lasting systems of support on their departure (see Chapter 8), fundamentally their influence was limited to the here and now of the hospital stay. It was not that the importance of the life contexts of patients was not recognized, or sympathized with, but rather that these were overwhelming and felt to be beyond scope—and the stakes were high.

Dr L's approach mirrors the dominant approach of the (relatively limited) international efforts to combat TB.[15] These have largely focused on efforts toward biomedical advances: the development of diagnostic methods with increased efficiency, specificity, or accuracy (and sometimes all of these); the development of less toxic, shorter TB treatment regimens that do not require a handful of drugs every day (plus some), especially for drug-resistant TB; and (as yet unsuccessful) efforts toward the development of a better TB vaccine, given that the Bacille Calmette-Guérin (BCG) vaccine is not regarded as highly effective in the long term.[16] These have contributed to substantive improvements in the experience of seeking treatment and the international burden of TB. At the same time, the focus on managing the TB microscopic pathogen can also obscure (or encourage us to forget) the macroscopic fact that TB was all but eradicated in Europe almost a century ago through the powerful tonic of improved living conditions. And, as all the stories in this chapter show us, what is left out in how the constitution of health is understood in biomedical settings is often what matters most in the experience of illness.

In noting that the foreclosure of experiences and stories is a standard part of the medical approach, I am not, then, diminishing the work of the health staff. The discussions that took place on the weekly joint doctors' medical rounds often had the feeling of a team trying to work out the image made by a pile of puzzle pieces, with the pile missing some pieces and including some from a different puzzle altogether. The difficulties involved in talking about substance use (mostly illegal, often judged) meant that it became a puzzle piece of unknown size, importance, frequency, and location. Uncertain disease etiology makes for uncertain biomedical treatment decisions, and when decisions are critical, the immediate arsenal of the hospital can be employed in the search for improved health, which remains in focus as the health care providers adaptively "tinker" (to use Anne-Marie Mol's term) with treatment, using the tools at their disposal in search of the best possible outcome.[17] The word "tinkering" has the right meaning, but it also has lightness to it that does not really express the burden of the process. Folders fatten with ongoing searches for answers. TB can be cured, say the posters on the wall of the hospital. It can also kill. Treatment decisions carry the very real weight of a potential body in a coffin and the spread of pathogens across populations. The question then becomes how to foster a different approach that meets the needs of health care providers and patients alike.

SYNDEMICS AND CO-CONSTITUTING HEALTH FORCES

In exploring the dynamic between TB and substance use, my work relates to a substantial body of literature focused on the synergistic interaction between diseases or health conditions (commonly referred to as comorbidities or co-occurrences in biomedicine) and the ways in which this is seated within social relations. The theory most widely applied in this work, syndemics, has been spearheaded by Singer and influentially defined as "the concentration and deleterious interaction of two or more diseases or other health conditions in a population" as a consequence of "social inequity and the unjust exercise of power" (2009, 226). The concept of syndemics has gained popularity and been drawn upon and adapted by a wide variety of fields, and as it has done so, it has taken on various emphases and forms, but in this definition (one of the earlier ones), the concept emphasizes the ways that health conditions develop within, and as consequence of, historical processes and life contexts. While it may be possible to isolate causative disease pathogen, the power of the pathogen to "make sick" is shaped by circumstance.[18] Here the definition also draws attention to the ways that health conditions can develop symbiotically, be reliant on each other for development, or change each other's course. For example, Felicity's early onset of neurosyphilis symptoms and Babalwa's TB were most likely related to their untreated HIV infections. The mental health challenges they faced, though unspoken, must also be regarded as a product of these synergies.

As others have shown, syndemic theory also valuably highlights how health conditions can interact synergistically to become something greater than the sum of their parts (Weaver and Mendenhall 2014; Engelmann and Kehr 2015). Mutually present diseases may not continue to act as discrete entities; in synergy, they may result in a constellation of symptoms that fits into neither original disease category. (For example, the disseminated TB Babalwa experienced [TB that has spread from the initial site of infection in the lungs to elsewhere in the body] develops almost exclusively in immune-suppressed patients, such as those infected with HIV.) Disease distinctions frequently become blurred or even dissolve in dynamic interaction, and sometimes, something completely new is formed, upsetting diagnostic categories (Human 2011). These are important conceptual gains that have valuable practical implications for care provision, and the extent to which the concept of syndemics has resonated is evident in the increasing circle of disciplines in which it is used (Singer, Bulled, and Ostrach 2020; Singer et al. 2017) and the corresponding critiques (see, for example, Sangaramoorthy and Benton 2021).

Syndemics has been widely used to theorize the interaction between substance use and pathogenic diseases (Bhardwaj and Kohrt 2020), yet I have found that the concept does not meet the ethical or conceptual needs of my data. I have two key concerns, the first of which is that syndemic theory lends itself to the pathologization of substance use. In Chapter 2, I described the slippery ground of defining substance use (as a behavior) as a "condition," "disorder," or "disease" and how this is determined by moral determinations of substance as much—if not more—than lived experience or biological realities. Furthermore, the moral censure and stigma experienced by people who use substances can mean that admission of substance use can change the care received, influencing the path of TB disease even if that use is not classifiable (in technical terms) as a condition or disorder. Yet the fractious boundaries between use and "abuse" are generally not engaged with in the syndemics literature. Rather, the term "(ab)use" is employed without a critical discussion as to the normative assumptions, and moral sanction, this holds (see, for example, Singer 2000, 2006, 2012). Babalwa's story shows us the danger of this: in the substance use group, her drinking was, similarly, uncritically described as "abuse." This fixed whatever assaults her mental health was facing and her corresponding search for the solace in alcohol (in a place and a time where there was little solace to be found) into a pathology, and it allowed what really made her sick to slide into the realm of unimportance.

My second concern is that syndemic theory is increasingly undoing its own powerful work in blurring the boundaries between the common biomedicine distinctions between "the social" and "the medical." Though key elements of the term "syndemic" have remained fairly stable (most notably the focus on inequality as predisposing of poor health), Singer and colleagues have developed and adapted the term in numerous ways since early use.[19] Newer iterations of the concept lean toward making structural and life conditions "contextual" factors against which two or more known disease entities wrap into one another. This was not how the concept started. In his original work on the substance (ab)use, violence, "AIDS"[20] (shortened to the acronym SAVA) syndemic (2000, 2006), Singer focuses on the ways in which behaviors and life circumstances affect disease status. Here drug (ab)use is seen as one of interacting "conditions"; it is an arm of the syndemic interaction. However, in their explication of the

concept, Singer and Clair (2003) distinguish between a syndemic at a population level, described as "two or more epidemics interacting synergistically and
contributing as a result to an excess *disease* load in a population," and at an individual level, where it is described as "health consequences of the *biological interactions* that occur when two or more diseases or health conditions are co-present
in multiple individuals within a population" (emphasis added). If we are to
apply the emphasis on disease to the SAVA syndemic, it implies that the most
important role player—or public health concern—is AIDS, for this is the only
one that is, without question, defined as a disease of a biological nature, even if it
is affected by structural factors such as gender and class. In later work, substance
(ab)use changes location in syndemics descriptions: it becomes the context that
causes two (infectious) diseases to be in syndemic interaction (Singer 2014).
With the increasing emphasis on biological effects, there is slippage in the ways
in which life circumstances, experiences, and health conditions are represented;
structural conditions and life patterns become base cogs that increase the
chances of pathogenic diseases twisting into each other, resulting in biological
changes. Health and biology are made synonymous. This shrinking undercuts
some of the concept's capacity to blur the boundaries between that which is, in
biomedicine, regarded as "social" and that which is regarded as "biomedical."
This allows for a narrow focus on what it is that makes poor health and therefore
what is seen as necessary to make good health. It is, then, precisely in this
blurring—the reminder that health cannot be understood outside of life experiences, patterns, and context—that the term "syndemics" has most value.[21]

MUTUAL MASKING

I met Shireen in her third internment at DP Marais, a stay of four months. She
was thirty-five years old and a mother of four. After her discharge from the hospital, I sought her out at home, a one-roomed tin structure perched on a wind-
swept hill, overlooking the Indian Ocean. Hers was a life literally and figuratively
at the very margins of the city. The room-house was just fitted with a single bed,
a single white plastic chair, and a small cupboard. The door opened onto a view
of the communal toilet and taps. The small window was so high it only framed
blue sky. Shireen lived here with her youngest son and her husband. This was, by
her description, a step up from their living conditions prior to her recent hospital admission. The family's home had been a smaller, rougher shack, located in a
much more crowded settlement. They had been given the plot and materials to
build their home by the City of Cape Town during Shireen's illness.

Shireen explained that she had started smoking tik six years before. Prior to
this, her entertainment had come in the form of alcohol, but her husband, Henry,
preferred tik. When she was drunk and he was high, they fought, partly because

he would go to smoke with other women and this made her uncomfortable. In a bid for a smoother relationship, she switched substances. It was a strategic decision that worked, she said. Their fighting reduced and they used with care, always ensuring there was enough food in the house and only using at weekends and when together.

About two years into using tik, Shireen started coughing and struggling to breathe. She had asthma attacks that had Henry frequently calling an ambulance for emergency oxygen. Over the months that followed, she lost weight, lots of weight. When her gaunt frame was swallowed up by her clothing, she decided it was time to take action: she stopped smoking tik. However, after two weeks of abstinence, things were not looking much better, "I still looked like a person who was smoking, even though I wasn't," she explained. It was only then that she sought out health care beyond the emergency ambulance services. A TB diagnosis quickly followed.

The literature describes delayed treatment seeking in people who use drug as primarily related to stigma and negative health care responses (Gundersen, Yimer, and Bjune 2008). In Shireen's story, we see delayed treatment seeking and treatment interruption associated with substance use, but as she described, it was less related to stigma and more related to a different reading of her own body and symptoms due to the TB–substance use co-constitution. She had been experiencing most of the signs of TB—notably coughing, shortness of breath, weight loss, loss of appetite, and, eventually, night sweats. These are easily legible as likely evidence of TB among South Africans living in marginalized conditions. And yet Shireen did not read her symptoms as TB because substance use fore-fronted a different reading of her own body, and the symptoms she experienced could equally be read as signs of methamphetamine use, or in the case of night sweats, withdrawal. This meant that for a long time, she did not take action. Other people who used drugs explained that they assumed they felt sick because they were not using enough drugs because drugs are broadly experienced as a palliative to life's harsh realities and interpreted as a medicine of sorts. Consequently, when symptoms appeared, some people reported that they increased their intake, rather than seeking an alternative cause of being poorly. The signs of TB that can be so clear are rendered murky for people who use drugs.[22]

Co-constitutions demand and deserve our attention not only because of what they produce but also because of the ways in which they obscure and obfuscate cause and effect in the constitution of the health statuses for people affected and health care personnel alike.[23] In the TB–substance use co-constitution, clarity is particularly inhibited because conversations are inhibited by moral judgment and, for drugs, the pall of illegality. In this context, not knowing what can and should be said looms large. Choices become harder and are frequently made in and through doubt. Our attention should, I suggest, linger on that which is masked as much as that which is made. Both have ramifications for health and illness.

BRINGING LIFE CONDITIONS AND
EXPERIENCES TO THE FORE

To return to the beginning: Lucinda's intake interview reminds us that the ways that people affected by TB explain their illness is often not in terms of disease pathology, but rather in terms of life circumstances. This is not necessarily because they do not know that a pathogen is a necessary condition for their poor health, but rather because they have lived the ways that their TB illness has come to fruition. Such descriptions of TB disease source and course matter, because they hold an inherent truth that is too easily forgotten by TB health systems: biomedical innovations are needed because inequality prevails. At a minimum, then, health practitioners and researchers therefore have an ethical responsibility to ensure that they do not exacerbate this inequality, and one way to ensure this is not to pathologize life patterns.

Babalwa's life story, juxtaposed as it is with the way she was treated in the substance (ab)use group (and the way she berates herself), reminds us of the importance of holding the fullness (or emptiness) of life in view when we think about how health dispositions are constituted and how health forces wrap together. This not only shifts blame but also suggests that longer-term health requires thinking about necessary changes that lie outside of her body. Medical anthropologists have a responsibility to use our skills to bring the messiness of life into the scope and purview of health care providers in a way that allows for better care provision (Macdonald, Mason, and Harper 2019). (If anthropologists cannot suggest practical and productive ways for health care systems and providers to generate productive responses to health forces, expecting biomedical practitioners to do so seems beyond reason.) Syndemics steps us toward this, but at the same time, the theory has evolved to lean increasingly toward prioritizing a focus on interactions between diseases and conditions that result in biological changes, which encourages a pathologization of life patterns. What is really needed is a way of looking at the constitution of health dispositions that better encourages the recognition that life patterns are not simply "context" to illness; they may well be the critical health force making illness.

The hopelessness described by Dr L with regards to engaging with these broader issues is precisely because of the narrow biomedical approach of seeking to generate health through healing a physical body, rather than a person in the world.[24] Yet here, Babalwa is again illustrative. For though the way she was viewed in the substance (ab)use group was one-dimensional and the way she was represented in her records did no justice to her life experiences—as happened with some patients, especially those who had arrived desperately ill and required extensive care—she was in the hospital over an extended period and additional layers of knowing her (and caring about her) were constructed over time (sometimes against mandates). Babalwa was allowed to stay in the hospital as long as possible; she earned money through a laundry program supported by staff members, and she saved all she could from the government-provided disability grant she had accessed with hospital support. After her discharge, she was able to rent a small shack and reforge her family, with the help of the hospital social worker who had negotiated their return to her. She kept in touch with one of the occupational therapy team, who paid her occasionally to come in and clean her house. Reports were that she had her children back and was doing well. Had she been treated only as a body and not as a person in the world, I doubt this would have been the outcome of all the medical treatment she received.

4 · SALIENCE AND SILENCE
Data, Evidence, and the Making of Figure Facts

From an anthropological standpoint, scientific facts become significant in terms of how, in their partiality, they become incorporated into an on-going struggle for life.   —Adriana Petryna, *Life Exposed* (2013, 25)

MONITORING AND EVALUATION: COUNTING SUCCESS IN THE WORLD OF TB

Every year, the Global Tuberculosis Report is published by the WHO. The report provides an overview of progress toward internationally set goals for ending TB, internationally recommended approaches to prevention and treatment, the funding landscape, and key new research findings. It also details each country's estimated TB burden and the reported treatment statistics. This report is the most authoritative presentation of "figure facts," indicating which countries are facing the greatest challenges in terms of TB burden and which are succeeding in their response efforts. The Global Tuberculosis Report is not only an indicator of good governance and a matter of international honor and standing; it also provides evidence of which countries are in need and which are worthy of funding and assistance.

In each of the three clinics in which I conducted research, I was privy to the first line of the production of the monthly records that would eventually feed into the WHO Global Report. Every TB-related event or interaction, from simple symptom screening to a genetic test for a TB strain, needed documentation. Meeting set targets (number of people screened, tested, initiated on treatment, completing treatment, and cured) was a way of assessing not only the success of the TB program but also the individual worth and work of health care providers. Along with successes, each month, the number of people "lost to follow up"—those who had not completed treatment and could either not be found or not be made to complete treatment—was tallied. "Losing" people was easy enough if patients did not arrive at health care facilities. Patients often lived in informal housing areas, where homes were unmarked and hidden among a maze of others. Wary of having health care workers arrive at their homes in what might result in stigma and shame, patients sometimes provided incorrect home locations; cell phone numbers provided by patients frequently changed; and efforts to procure work meant that people frequently moved away. These patients slid off the books recording treatment progress and onto the registers of failure.

At each step of the TB care cascade, the numbers needed to show enough success. This meant attaining targets for the number of people screened, diagnosed, starting on treatment, completing treatment, and treated to "cure." This placed constant pressure on clinic staff because as much as these data were used to track patient progress, they were used to hold staff accountable, to check their "compliance" to the requirements of the job. Failure to attain required figures would reflect badly on everyone. If the numbers were below target, the community care workers risked the wrath of the nurse they worked under, who in turn risked the ire of the doctor in charge, who needed to demonstrate good numbers to the district coordinator, and so forth.

This tension torqued at the end of each quarter as teams tried to ensure that their numbers proved their worth. The challenges were not only related to performance. During our time in one clinic, my colleagues and I watched as the data entry staff and the TB clinic nurse wrestled with numbers that were not slotting into the monitoring and evaluation framework they were obliged to use. The resulting blank spaces on the forms indicated that the clinic was not attaining its goal of patients tested, maintained in treatment, and completing treatment. The TB sister blamed the data input officer, who explained, unsuccessfully, that the problem was that the format for data was not one that allowed an accurate input of data. "We must work harder!" said the sister in charge.

A few days later, my colleague and I arrived at the clinic to find both the sister and the treatment supporter threatening resignation. The clinic doctor, who visited twice weekly, was angry at the "poor" monthly figures. He was openly frustrated that the previous team working in TB, recently rotated to a different area in the clinic, had had much better results. Why could not they do as well? The implication was that they were inept or, at very least, lazy. To us, the treatment supporter lamented that what the doctor did not know (because they had not told him) was that the previous team had massaged the TB tracking data by excluding from the records people who use substances—experienced as the most unruly of patients and the least likely to complete treatment. This had resulted in the stellar results (and the certificate of achievement on the wall) the previous team had obtained.

Examining the historical development of the use of statistics in Europe, Porter (2012) shows how the pursuit of "cure rates" led to the development of mutable, suitable categories that constructed favorable (and exceedingly questionable) presentations of the efficacy of asylums in restoring mental health. Death "weighed" on cure rate statistics (2012, 589); the only hope for asylums for positive results where death could not be avoided was either to reject patients or to not classify people as patients of the institution. Porter calls the shaping of figures to purpose rather than reality "statistical opportunism" (2012, 590). In her examination of survey processes in demographic research in Malawi, Crystal Biruk refers to processes of "cooking" data, which involve, in part, the creation of data to suit the research purpose. Such opportunism and cooking seems to have been at play in the clinics in Cape Town, too, where staff experienced record-keeping as tyrannical.[1]

I never found out just how a portion of TB patients were hidden from view, whether through refusing people who used substances treatment or simply through recording their data elsewhere. Subsequent discussions with health care providers from other facilities have indicated that this clinic was not exceptional. I heard of shadow books in other clinics—records made by the TB clinic staff that were used to track patients but, somehow, kept outside of view of their superiors.[2] Whatever the system, the result was that—at least to some degree— records were hidden of people who used substances and had tuberculosis.

This chapter is about my own efforts at making the TB–substance use co-constitution numerically legible through a folder review in DP Marais Hospital. Those of us who tend to peddle in the power of narratives to illuminate and unsettle often find that our qualitative methods and findings are not taken seriously unless anchored by what I call "figure facts": numbers that are easy to grasp, which neatly serve as proof of an issue at hand, therefore circulate easily and galvanize action in a way that narrative evidence rarely does. I show how the figures I produced in DP Marais, to my surprise, served this purpose. Yet, though I stand by the figures I made, in this chapter I show that even when there is no (or limited) motivation for bias in the construction of numbers, morals, needs, and interpretations are folded into their construction. Numbers are never neutral, but we can make them better by developing and reading them in concert with ethnographic data.

A MATTER OF FIGURES

At my first visit to DP Marais, I heard from the hospital staff that approximately 70 percent of patients in the hospital at any given time were substance (ab) users.[3] This estimate seemed remarkably, if not implausibly, high. At the time the substance use–TB co-constitution was largely unwritten in South African litera-ture. Only one article focused on it directly and that related to alcohol use (Peltzer et al. 2012). The hospital's mandate was ultimately to care for people in "medical" need—those too sick to take their medication at home. The necessary condition for admission was TB, and the likely condition was HIV seropositiv-ity. Substance use was seen, as I described in the previous chapter, as an overtly "social" issue and therefore not directly in the hospital purview.

Yet as my research progressed, this figure became easier to believe. Substance (ab)use was mentioned casually, in everyday ways, in conversation among patients. "Pull on it like it's a tik lolly!" explained one patient, sounding exasperated, when another patient, a young woman, was not succeeding in inhaling on her asthma pump correctly and was starting to panic. Substance-using patients were frequent topics of conversation between staff. "What do you expect of a druggie?" asked one nurse of another in discussion about a patient who was found to be sleeping on a mattress that was thickly layered with sheets and towels she had surreptitiously been gathering from the hospital to sell on her departure. But it was difficult to tell to what degree the conversations and the estimated figure of 70 percent were a genuine reflection of levels of substance use in hospitalized patients and to what degree the illicit nature of substance use and moral judgments attached to it resulted in the talk and an exaggerated estimation.

Intrigued, I selected a date in April—long enough after Christmas for the holiday period not to affect the patient numbers and before the winter rains that always resulted in an influx of people who lived on the street and were more likely to use substances. I set about conducting a cross-sectional folder review of all the patients in the hospital on that one day. Each patient had a dedicated ring-bound folder that held patient records on drug regimes, nutritional intake, and medical tests. These were accompanied by referral letters and all notes from the doctors, the physiotherapist, the psychologist, the social workers, the occupational therapist, and, where applicable, the HIV nurse and her team of assistants. (The nurses kept their daily records separately.) Folders were portioned into sections for these different intervention areas, marked by colored card. Notes were made and read by all the clinical staff, although it was the nurses and doctors who used the folders most as they kept track and communicated (with each other and across shift changes) about key tracking and matters to attend to. In the acute wards, the folders lay readily accessible on tables at the ends of beds that were contoured, but never filled, by the blanketed and often sleeping, angular bodies of very sick patients. Here they were accessible for everyday use (the sicker the patient, the more frequent the use). In other wards, folders were stored in the nurses' offices, to be set out when the doctors were due to do their rounds.

Out of the 179 patients in the hospital at the time, I was able to review 176 folders; the other three were lost, not to be refound, somewhere in the hospital system. Of these, 167 folders contained some information relating to substance use,[4] my key area of focus (and therefore my N). As I shifted through the files, I noted down any reference to substance use in detail, while also recording other areas, such as gender, age, referral institutions—anything, really, that I thought might shed light on the TB–drug use co-constitution. I then coded and tabulated all the information into one, expansive data sheet.

This slow and tedious process resulted in one particularly useful figure. Time and again, people I was speaking to would express surprise (and sometimes disbelief, if they did not work directly in the realm of TB) that there was a notable overlap, or interaction, between TB and substance use. My reply gained fluency with repetition: "26% of the patients in DP Marais TB Hospital were using tik, heroin, or mandrax at the time of becoming ill with TB." Numbers, or figures, have an easy authority (Porter 1996), and the fact that over a quarter of the hospital patients should be using what are—in common perception—"hard" (or addictive) drugs served as satisfyingly incontrovertible evidence that I was onto something. Yet, while I stand by this figure, I also know—because I went through the painstaking process of making it—that this figure says as much about my own perceptions and opinions and those of the folder-fillers and note-takers as it does about the people in the hospital.

SEARCHES FOR "TRUTH"

In evidence-based medicine, randomized controlled trials (RCTs) provide the gold standard of data production. RCTs are large-scale studies, in which people are randomly selected to receive or not receive a particular intervention. Their health status is then statistically measured before and after the intervention is implemented. The design and implementation structure of RCTs is ultimately aimed at presenting the structure of "truth," or the reality that emerges when bias has been stripped away. RCTs play a critical role in knowledge production, but the results they produce, and numbers more broadly, are never neutral (Erikson 2012; Stevenson 2014; Jain 2013). In order to measure human behavior and experience, complex life worlds need to be trimmed down to measurable "data points" (Adams 2013, 86). This is not a straightforward process. Decisions have to be made about classificatory slots that define what is measured. More decisions have to be made about how to extract the desired data points, or measurables, from the context within which they exist. Determinations have to be made about when those data points are extracted or whether a data point does not meet the needs of the classificatory slot set out. Layers of interpretation must then go into cleaning the data, deciding what to calculate, and how to interpret the results. Choices have to be made about the presentation (or nonpresentation) of the outcomes. These work processes all occur in moral and political worlds; notions of what is good and what is necessary infuse every step; research has to be funded, and with money comes vested interests. Yet these important shaping influences and power dynamics are rarely fully acknowledged (Brives, Le Marcis, and Sanabria 2016).

Not only are the results not neutral, they are also partial. RCTs can only measure what is categorized in the research design, stifling the possibilities for the emergence of new forms of knowledge (Adams 2013) and framing what comes to be classified as true (Venkat 2016). In this, RCTs build present assumptions about what is true into the "facts" of the future in what Brives and colleagues (2016) call "anticipatory politics." Categorization processes require that attention to small-scale life details is set aside, that individuals and their circumstances get subsumed into the masses, and that those who do not fit neatly into the set of classifications are rendered invisible (Biehl 2005). Beyond this, RCTs seek to control for the effects of factors outside of those immediately measured. Context has to be ignored, rather than engaged with, in a process Brives and colleagues (2016) have described as "strategic unknowing." But context, as I show below, matters. Not only does it shape the emerging results, but it also determines the relevance of those results.

FOLDER REVIEW REVEAL

The problems I have set out above do not nullify the fact that "how much" or "how many" of something can really matter. The collated figures showed that the alcohol use of over half (54 percent) of all patients was considered "problematic" by hospital staff. Almost 20 percent had alcohol use levels noted as high in their files and a further 34 percent had some indications that staff interpreted their alcohol use levels as high. Forty percent of patients were recorded as smoking cigarettes, just under a quarter were recorded as smoking dagga, and over a fifth (22 percent) as smoking tik. Mandrax use was recorded for 10.8 percent of all patients, and 2.4 percent had heroin use recorded.[5] As elsewhere, men were generally recorded as having higher levels of use than women, although this was not the case for tik in people with drug-sensitive TB, where—counter the trends in the treatment center data—more women (23 percent) than men (19 percent) were recorded as using tik.[6]

My figure fact (26 percent) suggested a particular kind of a problem, partly because I was trading on the assumptions of a particular kind of behavior attached to the substances I included in the count. An alternative collated figure, including cigarette and alcohol use, shows a total of 77 percent of all patients using any substances. Excluding cigarettes (because the social acceptability of cigarette use meant that it was not generally tied to notions of abuse, despite the well-established tobacco-TB co-constitution), a total of 71 percent of patients were substance (ab)users. Viewed this way, the 70 percent estimation by doctors and staff was remarkably accurate. However, if, in addition to excluding cigarettes, mild alcohol use was excluded, this figure still shows that almost half (47.9 percent) of patients were using substances when they became sick with TB. These numbers and their variations tell us two key things: substance use and TB did seem to be co-constituting for patients in DP Marais. How the extent of this co-constitution is assessed is dependent on how (ab)use is understood. In the hospital as elsewhere, this was an extremely subjective determination.

MINING FOLDERS, MAKING FACTS

Substance use was unusual in that information about it was collected by a range of staff—it was everybody's problem. Information about an individual's patterns of substance use was generally first collected by a doctor doing the intake clerking procedures.[7] As part of this process, a "social history" would be elicited, including home and family circumstances and some information about substance use. The exact structure of the data recorded in files from intake interviews differed between the doctors, and the tone of communication—in relation to substance use at least—was generally one of pragmatism, sometimes leaning toward terseness. Some doctors would gather detailed information, substance by substance. Others would ask a general question about alcohol and drug use; follow up on information offered, if any; and let the silences be. This intake interview provided information on potential contraindications between medication and substances, and it indicated the chances that withdrawals—current or imminent—would need to be pharmaceutically managed. For patients who acknowledged regular use, this initial interview also hinted at chances of the patient "absconding" from the hospital, as I discuss below.

Subsequently, but generally within the first two weeks of hospitalization, other members of the staff tasked with providing support (much of it classed "social") for patients in the hospital did their own assessments. Wendy, the substance (ab)use coordinator, used an adapted version of a standard four-question assessment for alcohol (ab)use to decide whether an individual would be called to the substance (ab)use groups; the social workers would gather more detailed information about family support, housing, and financial status;[8] the physiotherapist, dietician, and occupational therapists would all do their rounds, adding to the papers proliferating in the folders. This meant that the information I sought was spread across forms in the files. Information also varied in structure, detail, and quality, sometimes with content discrepancies, often subtle, such as slightly discrepant dates of illness onset, for example, perhaps a result of different interpretations of patient descriptions. Sometimes too there were overt contradictions; in one location in a file, the patient might be recorded as being HIV negative, and in another area, there would be detailed history of HIV treatment processes. These discrepancies happened because each staff member gathering data acted from their personal and professional perspectives and purposes, and from the differences in the information notes, it appeared that they did not necessarily look at what their colleagues had recorded.

Subjectivities shaped the records and were particularly obvious in relation to alcohol use and determinations of whether this was or was not "abuse." Dr M, the Ward 5 doctor, tended to rely on the occupational therapy team to ask about substance use, though he did not always agree with their findings. An AA affiliate, Wendy was overtly in favor of abstinence and was quick to note any alcohol consumption as problematic. As an older, respected woman of dignified stature who spoke with a comfortable authority, her view influenced others on the occupational therapy team. Dr M was concerned that this labeling might pathologize cultural and social practices of traditional beer drinking. In one planning meeting for newly arrived MDR patients, discussion turned, not for the first time, to "different drinking styles," and Dr M commented that some of his patients only drank "casually," suggesting that this alcohol consumption did not necessarily indicate disruptive drunkenness. "They all drink casually!" replied Wendy, implying that "casual" was either a thinly veiled admission of "heavy drinking" or indicative of the denial that she saw as a characteristic of addiction. Dr M countered, saying some were just drinking [African] beer with their friends—passing the bucket round the circle, as was a cultural norm. "Beer has alcohol in it!" Soraya, the occupational therapist, shot back, with a hint of a laugh cushioning a greater tone of exasperation. Soraya was not so much asserting that the problem was the patient's misrepresentation of use (although she generally agreed with Wendy), but, as someone whose religious beliefs disallowed alcohol consumption, she saw alcohol consumption per se as negative, no matter how much was consumed. These differences meant that it was difficult to know whether substance use noted as "abuse" in the folders was genuinely disruptive or simply assumed to be so.

The contradictions—subtle and overt—were not just about staff subjectivities. My discussions with patients indicated that they knew—or at least suspected—that how they were viewed by hospital personnel could affect the institutional care and support they would receive—from hospital length stay, to disability grants, to family meetings. This meant that there was value for patients in crafting narratives (or silences) to best meet their needs. For example, a patient might indicate that they were experiencing challenges with alcohol use at home as a way of encouraging the staff to extend their stay but would deny using tik, which was actually the substance they used regularly. This was because tik use was more stigmatized and might result in additional, uncomfortable surveillance.

Sometimes the way patients assessed what narrative to provide depended on who was asking and how that asking was being done. Many nurses came from the same neighborhoods as the patients they treated, which likely inhibited admissions of substance use because stories can (and did) traverse the hospital complex boundaries. At the same time, nurses suggested that they often had an insider view. There was little hiding to be done in the open wards they oversaw, and their shared backgrounds set up places of comfort with patients, in contrast to . . . with the doctors. Speaking of Felicity's reluctance to admit substance use (see Chapter 3), one nurse explained, "She admitted [substance use] afterwards, but not in front of the doctor. Sometimes the patient is scared . . . then afterwards they will come and tell you this and that . . . I always remind them . . . that this is your doctor, you can speak to them. But sometimes I think, the word 'Doctor' for [people from our community], it is like, you don't say anything [to the doctor] in the communities. So that's why sometimes they open up more to us."

The ways in which patients described their substance use also changed in what I call "disclosure creep"; an initial denial of substance use changed to an admission of some substance use, which evolved to acknowledgment of regular and disruptive substance use. This creep depended on a lack of (overt) negative response to each subsequent admission. Sometimes this process took months, and other times, it occurred gradually in one interaction, as happened in a focus group I ran with a group of eight women patients in the hospital. In the beginning, women said they only drank on weekends (and one woman, Maggie, said she only drank socially). I asked when the weekend started. Someone said Friday, which was corrected by another woman to Thursday, to general agreement. Then, Lydia pointed out that any other holiday was also regarded as a day for drinking. "And over Christmas, drunk the whole time!" she said. Then I asked, "What if, in the week (by now truncated to Monday to Wednesday), a friend comes round with a case [of beer]?" The answer was that that is okay for drinking, too.[9] It slowly emerged that there never was a time that was off-limits for drinking. As one admission in the focus group was not judged, the next was acceded, to the accompaniment of much laughter. In the laughter was the common (and perhaps relieved) recognition that they had each withheld information, perhaps for fear of judgment between each other, or by me and my research assistant. Other times, disclosure was not from the patient themselves but from conversations with the referring clinic (which would perhaps be recorded in folders), from other patients (which would be included in conversations, excluded from folders), or because they were seen to be associating in the hospital with another patient, who was more revealing about their use.

Other times, people changed what they revealed, because their desire to stay in the hospital changed over time. With extended stays, patients came to know which narratives were most likely to provide the outcome they were seeking. If, for example, on arrival a patient feared that admitting substance use would negatively influence their stay, they might deny this, but on later discovering that substance use could be a reason for extending the hospital stay (for those patients submitting to hospital authority), use might be revealed. If hospitalization had seemed appealing at first but was losing its luster, being caught using substances was a quick way to ensure an early departure.

In his classic text on "illness narratives," Arthur Kleinman (1988) suggested that the stories people tell about their illness are sense-making, explanatory tools for patients and therefore worthy of attention. In the hospital, illness narratives are not only sense-making tools, but also life-making tools, differently crafted and used by the same person at different times, depending on the perceived power and role of the person to whom they were talking (see also Briggs and Mantini-Briggs 2003). Patients were not desperately trying to make sense of a confusing world; they were actively navigating a world of limited resources.

ANCHORING THE FIGURE FACTS

The consequence of these uncertainties was that in mining the folders, as I crystallized complex webs of information into organized, quantifiable categories,

I consciously selected what I decided to be the most likely truth-reflection. (Or, as in the case of employment, I simply excluded the collected data from analysis.) Sometimes this relied on personal knowledge of the people who had recorded the information. (Staff member A, for example, would classify any alcohol use as abuse, whereas staff member B would only indicate "abuse" if the patient themselves had indicated dependence on alcohol.) Sometimes it simply required that I looked across categories in files to reconcile impossible discrepancies or similarities. Here I applied a hierarchy of trust—if the medical records indicated ART provision, but the social worker records said HIV negative, I ignored the latter. I could never quite be sure that repetition and consistency in the material in the folders were accurate reports. I had no proof whether the source of repetition was the patient, who provided the same information to each staff member, or whether staff had reviewed each other's inputs and replicated information.

Epidemiological research studies have inbuilt mechanisms to try to eliminate, or at least reduce, subjectivities in data. But subjectivities will always lurk in data and—as others (Bourgois 2002; Béhague, Gonçalves, and Victora 2009) have suggested—there is value in the integration of ethnographic and epidemiological studies, not least because ethnography can explain the subjectivities that remain.

Yet preexisting data may be all that is available due to time, resources, or ethical constraints, and it tends to have more gaps, repetitions, and inconsistencies. Here the ethnographer has a different role: to layer interpretations (Hacking 1990). Ethnographic knowledge allows one to craft the available data so that the numbers produced at the end are the most likely "truth." Reading the resultant numbers through ethnography provides another important layer of clarity. This was particularly evident for the rates of heroin use (2 percent), which emerged in my review.

ZINTLE/INAM

Zintle arrived at DP Marais from the large tertiary public hospital close to the city center. She had been admitted there wracked with TB, on the verge of death; she was started on TB treatment and referred to DP Marais. Her referral declared her as someone who used substantial amounts of heroin ("Heroin abuser +++"). A few weeks of TB treatment turned Zintle's health around. Soon she was chirpily joining in the women's occupational therapy sessions. Petite and muscular (she had once belonged to a women's road cycling team), she had the habit of calling me "Baby" (no accidental "doctor" for her) and would pop into my room regularly for a chat or simply to seek some sympathy for the pain of damaged nerves, likely from HIV, but also possibly related to years of heroin use. One morning, she arrived in my office and announced, "Baby, my name is not Zintle."

Inam explained that she had been admitted to the tertiary hospital multiple times for pneumonia and, each time, slipped away without formal discharge. On her last admission, she had worried that if the administrators linked her person to her hospital folder, she would be turned around at the door, and so she supplied a different name that, inscribed in medical records, traveled with her to DP Marais. However, to access a government-provided disability grant, which, at about $100 per month, provided a neat nest egg on departure for those who stayed the course in the hospital and saved as they did so, the social workers needed Inam's national identity document (ID). This persuaded Inam to confess her deception. The confession, she said, was a relief; she was tired of getting called by a name that wasn't her own, and other patients had started to look suspiciously at her when she did not respond to her own name.

Weeks after her arrival, Inam was in the large room where women did ironing while we were discussing some impending discharges. "I am scared of leaving," Inam said. Did she expect to leave soon, I asked. With an overt expression of horror, she said, "I've only just arrived!" But soon after, Inam was dropped by the hospital transport at the home of an aunt, much earlier than planned. Rumors had leaked that Inam was selling drugs on the hospital premises. These had drowned any chances of an extended stay. Some weeks later, I called Inam's aunt. A day after arriving, Inam had "jumped" from home, likely, thought her aunt, to return to life on the streets, under a bridge. With months still to go, we both feared that Inam's chances of completing treatment and finding health were low. "It is hard . . ." whispered her aunt as we said goodbye.

In contrast with other substances (mandrax—11 percent, tik—21 percent), rates of heroin use in the hospital seem so low as to barely merit attention. But this was not the case. Rather, my 2 percent figure missed key facts; it did not capture the rates of people using heroin who came to the hospital (and made untimely departures) or the concern and consternation related to heroin use. In DP Marais, people who were known to use heroin were regarded as the ultimate "revolving door" patients. They frequently took leave of the hospital without permission, generally over the chain-link fence[10] and often within the first few days. When I extracted the numbers of early leavers from the hospital over a four-month period from hospital records, a slightly different picture emerged. In total, twenty-seven patients had either absconded or signed "red tickets" (forms indicating that the patient has chosen to leave without the doctor's consent) between January and April 2015. Of the twenty-four folders I was able to access, 92 percent ($n = 22$) had indications of use of high levels of alcohol and/or use of tik, mandrax, or heroin in their folders. Of these patients, 23 percent ($n = 5$) had records of heroin use.[11]

The chances of an early departure were seen to be so high that staff would sometimes hold off on doing a full "clerk" until the patient had stayed in the hospital for a day or two so as not to waste time on a patient who might quickly disappear. When I asked Dr N about a particularly disheveled new older female patient, she explained that the patient was addicted to heroin and "the only reason she hasn't jumped yet is because she is too sick." Patients who were not "clerked" did not have folders for me to review and did not even enter into the count.

Absconding was not necessarily because the patient had not wanted to come to the hospital. One referral letter read: "Patient has [no fixed address], on heroin, previous defaulter but requested admission and detox. Has been very compliant [to TB medication] since start of treatment." The same patient "jumped" the day after arriving. Substitution therapy such as methadone, which would lessen the misery of sudden withdrawal from heroin and has been shown to increase TB treatment completion in people who use heroin (Morozova, Dvoryak, and Altice 2013; Gupta et al. 2014; Bruce et al. 2014), was not available in secondary hospitals such as DP Marais. Even in copious amounts, the sedative diazepam was a poor substitute, especially in the open wards where discomfort was a public matter. Sometimes, staying in the hospital was just too hard.

Patients who used heroin also garnered attention in the hospital because they had reputations (fairly or not) for dishonesty and theft. They were regarded warily, and often treated with some reluctance, by staff. "I don't trust heroin users until you have proved yourself trustworthy" was the warning line that Dr L gave patients coming into the hospital whose heroin use was disclosed (either by themselves or through the referral letter), further reducing incentive to stay in the hospital. If we read the 2 percent figure describing the percentage of people in the hospital using heroin, in light of the ethnographic data, it is evident that this is indicative of the people who had the fortitude to stay in the hospital, despite challenging conditions, not the number of people who used heroin who came to the hospital.

CONCLUSION

Folder reviews are broadly considered the least scientific means of making numbers (Adams 2013), and yet the DP Marais figures I produced seemed to gain their own momentum, claiming leverage in a way that narratives of people who used substances in the hospital simply did not. Just after I produced the figures presented here, in 2014, they were circulated through provincial government structures. In 2015, they were used by a representative of the Province of the Western Cape in a presentation to the Central Drug Authority (South Africa's national drug body). I was also approached by a nonprofit organization (TB HIV Care) that works closely with government structures, to assist with piloting a response in DP Marais Hospital, and the small project we developed became one of the five priority projects of the Provincial Department of Health that year. The figures I produced made the fact of the relation between TB and substance use real, legible, and pressing. They reinforced Adia Benton's (2012) claim that descriptive processes of enumeration that do not attain the perceived "gold standard" of the randomized controlled trials still tend to carry greater authority than purely qualitative data sources or "vernacular accounts."

My project in describing how these data were made and how I extracted them from their context shows that even these—the most basic of figures—did not simply reveal themselves or could have emerged as unambiguous fact.

The neat and concrete numbers I have presented are best understood as created through multiple finding, filtering, and layering processes. As Biruk (2018) argues—all numbers are, to some degree, "cooked." This "cooking" happened at manifold levels: patient, health care provider, and researcher. Moreover, they are best understood in concert and conversation with ethnographic data. Theodore Porter (2012) writes that numbers engender trust because they are used to contain (as in, constrain) subjectivity. Here I have conducted an ethnography of the facts I brought into being. I have sought to show that when this is done carefully, subjectivities can compound in ways that stabilize understood truths into facts that are more, rather than less, "true," or valid, to use the statistical term.

Brives and colleagues (2016) have described the active ignoring of complexity that occurs in the design and implementation of RCTs as "strategic unknowing." The same can be said for the bureaucratic processes of recordkeeping where, similarly, the ways that people, relationships, and circumstances are recorded, crafts particular and partial images of reality. In this, numbers and bureaucracies are both regimes of power. In global health, this is not just about states exerting power over citizens, but also about global health power exerting itself over states.

What I have described in this chapter is a contrasting form of "strategic knowing." Nested in ethnographic data, we see, for example, that the levels of alcohol use are subject to debate, and the low levels of heroin use indicated in the hospital data do not necessarily indicate that there are few people who used heroin who become sick with TB. In the chapter that follows, I turn to explaining the reasons for the numbers that emerged relating to substance use in hospitalized patients, through exploring the social dynamics that shape who goes to DP Marais and why they do so.

5 · THE CHALLENGE OF
"UNRULY" PATIENTS

THEY DON'T DO A THING
FOR THEIR OWN HEALTH

There were six women in the room. Sister D, the nursing sister, was just start-ing her rotation in the TB section of the clinic. She was newly, and nervously, in charge. Mila, the "TB supporter," was responsible for patients taking their treatment in the clinic, following up on patients who had not appeared at the clinic, and overseeing DOTS supporters.[1] The four DOTS supporters—Lettie, Bronwyn, Sylvia, and Carol—were responsible for ensuring that every patient under their remit received and took medication daily "in community" until course completion. The DOTS supporters were all mature women, heavy set as a result of poor diets rather than abundant living.

Mila led the meeting. File by file, the group discussed each of the forty-three patients for whom they oversaw their daily pill consumption. Mila checked on each patient's progress by linking the file records with the recent reports made by the DOTS supporters. Where treatment was proceeding according to plan, the next sputum sample date for the patient was noted and Mila would hand a small sputum collection jar to the assigned DOTS supporter. Where treatment was not proceeding smoothly, discussions ensued. It did not take long for frus-trations about patients to be tumbling and churning in the room. As voices over-laid each other, I could not find a clear form to the discussion. But the shape of the frustrations became clear.

Carol spoke of Jasmine, a young woman who she said was frequently "*smoor dronk*" (blind drunk) and who disappeared for days each month after she received her disability grant. This explained the regular gaps on her treatment card that stretched into days. "They are flippin' drinking their money!" com-plained Bronwyn.

Carol had another "missing link," as they termed patients whose treatment cards were not filled with neat rows of tick marks indicating regular treatment.

He was a young man who had disappeared when the recent spate of shootings had started in their area. She could not find him, and even his parents did not know where he was. He was, she said, using drugs.

Sister D spoke of a young woman, Tilly, who had come in at the time of her scheduled clinic appointment the day before. But her patience was not enough to carry her through the required waiting period, and she had left before Sister D was ready to see her. Sylvia commented on Tilly, describing her as "once beautiful," but now "spaghetti thin . . . worse than spaghetti thin, vermicelli thin!" In commenting on Tilly's thinness, she was suggesting lost beauty, which was a common way of indicating drug use in women (Versfeld 2012).

Lettie, sensing that she might need to explain the frustrations in the room, turned to my colleague and me. "Drugs," she said, "are the biggest problem we have. . . ."

Sylvia, brimming with emotion, let loose a volley of woes. There was a house where most of the adults were using tik. A number of the children—and perhaps adults, though this was unclear—were in Sylvia's charge for their TB medication. Their parents' drug-induced negligence, she said, made it hard for her to ensure their treatment. The matter was complicated and distress heightened by the fact that Sylvia's daughter and grandchildren were residents in the house. Someone said that it was so much easier to work with children than it was to work with adults; with children, one just needed to build rapport. Someone else said it is best to work with old people.

Sister D, seemingly talking to everyone and no one in particular, suddenly exclaimed, "That's why the children are getting TB!" She explained, to growing attention from others in the room, that the previous day, she had received a call from Groote Schuur Hospital about a household where the children were all getting TB. A six-month-old baby had just been diagnosed positive. The hospital had called her and asked her to investigate. She had just realized that these children were in the house Sylvia was lamenting. "They'll all get sick!" Sister D said, adding that one of the adults had MDR TB.

"They make you sick . . . I am sick of the drugs!" opined Sylvia. The sickness she was referring to was not related to a pathogen; it was a "sickness" of frustration and stress caused by trying to provide TB care for people using drugs. "The problem with the drugs is that they are more important than the TB, and then, when they look like skeletons, Sister [D] must jump and send them to DP Marais," said Lettie.

One statement, made by Sister D toward the end of the meeting, explained the core of the frustrations. "*We* must answer because *they* are not compliant. I struggle to get sputum from them, then Doctor wants to know why they are not compliant, and they don't do a thing for their own health!"

Where does responsibility for TB cure lie? Does it lie with the patient, or patients? Does it lie with the health care system, with individual health care workers, or with the families of the sick? What happens when the person with

TB does not play the role of a compliant patient or does not want to be a patient? Who is rendered vulnerable, and in what ways, when TB treatment is not successful? And who is responsible then? How do the answers to these questions change when a TB patient also uses substance?

In this chapter, I turn to some of these questions. I show that the high levels of the TB–substance use co-constitution in DP Marais, presented in the last chapter, are not demonstrative of general levels of this co-constitution in the areas that feed patients to the hospital. Nor are these levels purely a result of the ways that substance use exacerbates illness severity. Rather, DP Marais has become a holding space for people who use substances because of the ways in which vulnerability, responsibility, and care come into tension in the TB response in Cape Town. In the previous chapter, I showed how health care workers are encouraged to send patients who use substances to DP Marais due to the current ways in which TB care is set up and success is measured, as well as the ways in which they are held accountable for numerical targets. Here I show how families and households appeal for state protection when they feel at risk from someone who is (potentially) infectious, and individuals themselves may request admission when they see admission as their best available option. The result is that the hospital is situated in a very particular way in relation to the TB–substance use co-constitution—and to people who use drugs and their families.

NOT FIT FOR DOTS: UNRULY PATIENTS

Bessie sat in the passage of the TB clinic waiting her turn to see Sister D after providing a sputum sample. She was small, thin, and folded into herself. The impression I had was that she was hoping the chair would swallow her whole before she was called into the consulting room. On the other side of the consulting room door, Sister D and Mila discussed the best plan for her treatment. They scoured her file. She was HIV positive and on ART, on TB treatment for drug-sensitive TB, and, in their language, a "defaulter." "They come in here and they are *so* sick," said Mila, "and they are always in a hurry. There is something chasing them . . . I think it is the drugs chasing them." As she filled in the paperwork to accompany the sputum sample Bessie had just provided, Mila hesitated, "I don't know what to fill in because she is defaulting. . . ." The forms were structured so as to record that treatment taking was, at least to some degree, regular. They did not allow for the complex stop–start trajectory of Bessie's treatment history.

Ten minutes later, Sister D called Bessie into the consulting room. She told Bessie that she would try to get her into DP Marais. It will be better for her, Sister D explained. (It would be better for them, too, but this she did not say.) She admonished Bessie, saying that she was also required to take care of her own health. "You are only getting worse, you're not going to get any better . . . you need to realize [this]. I now need to start everything from the beginning, because it is now four months that you have not been receiving treatment. . . . You are still you, only twenty-seven years old, but you will die!"

A day later, Bessie returned for her doctor's appointment. Her hunched-over posture still emanated hopelessness, or perhaps just the wish for invisibility, but she was neatly dressed and her hair was smoothed back and held fast with an Alice band. Above the thin paper mask all patients are required to wear in TB clinic waiting rooms, her eyes crinkled lightly in the shy smile of a greeting when she saw me. Dr P went to fetch her sputum results. These were positive; Bessie was confirmed to have TB (again). She must have suspected as much, for in response, she said that she had found someone willing to care for her children while she was away. Could she go to DP Marais? Her request was met by a warning: If she failed to complete her treatment once more, she would get terribly ill and there would be nothing more they could do. They would call DP Marais today and try to get her a bed. It would be much better for there here, but she would have to start her treatment right away. Threat, promise, and requirement intertwined—with hope pinned on hospital admission.

Dr P's warning—that they would be able to do nothing more if she failed to complete treatment once more—alluded to the possible consequence of repeated treatment interruption—the development of drug-resistant TB. He may also have been suggesting that he would be unwilling to keep treating her if she interrupted or stopped treatment again. Doctors constantly balanced concerns with the patients developing drug resistance through repeat treatment cessation, which was then transmissible to others, with the ethical imperative of providing treatment to the person in front of them. When drug use was present and seen as the reason for erratic treatment taking, health care provider decisions sometimes fell toward refusing further treatment for an individual, unless they acquiesced to hospital admission. This was set out in the referral letter for the admission of a young woman into DP Marais. "Tik abuser. Defaulter of note. Other family members on TB treatment—all retreatments. Dr V recommended no treatment unless admitted."[2] The place of tension the health care providers were inhabiting here was the pull of the right to health, on the one side, and, on the other side, the concern that they, the doctors, would be contributing to the development of drug-resistant TB, transmissible to others.

Bessie and the patients referred to in the opening vignette were what I call "unruly" patients. Unruly patients drank and/or used drugs. They exhibited a vexed relationship to the care they were being offered. In the framing of health care providers, these patients did not take treatment as prescribed, or not with trustworthy regularity, and so remained infectious, a danger to those around them, and a problem for their proof of work. They expected health care providers to respond to pleas for help when they had not responded to these health care providers' prior offers and efforts. Histories of treatment interruption did not fit with the structured requirements of recordkeeping. How was one to classify her treatment trajectory on the sputum bottle and the accompanying form? Further, these patients did not bode well for the requirements of future records.

Unruly patients are the opposite of the imagined, ideal, "good patient." Good patients took care of themselves and sought health care and attention without being unnecessarily demanding. These were the patients for whom the forms and recordkeeping processes were designed. They waited patiently for treatment in the clinic or attention in the hospital, accepted the treatment prescribed, and continued, until told to stop. They accepted some treatment side effects (orange urine, skin rashes, dizziness, and—commonly discussed among patients— terrifying nightmares) and asked about the others. They noted and followed the dates inscribed on clinic cards and came to and left the hospital when advised. Good patients were in control of life enough—but not too much—so as to be submissive to the health care system. They did not drink, did not use drugs. Good patients made the figure (75 percent) of people who are successfully treated for TB, or if not, it was the consequence of a medical puzzle, a "complex case." No one was deemed to be at fault.

Cheryl Mattingly (2014) has written about how the "good life" is a life worth living through, and despite, hardships and trials. Similarly, a "good patient" was a patient worth treating, despite complexities, because they were responsive to the biomedical advice given. Unruly patients, in contrast, were a trial to treat. Uncontained, they put their own lives and the health of their families at risk, and they undermined health care providers' efforts to do their jobs as required. Unruly patients were more likely to be sent by health care workers to DP Marais than patients of similar socioeconomic standing who did not use substances.[3] Sending them to the hospital was one way of removing troublesome patients from patient records, without the requirement of shadow books. This is certainly not to say health care workers were entirely self-interested. Frustration did not nullify care or hopes for patients' healing. Beyond this, there was the ever-present concern for family and household members at risk of infection ("They will all get sick!"). Sometimes efforts to protect families were directly in response to petitions from family members themselves. I turn to this next.

APPEALS FOR PROTECTION

Appeal 1: "He Has the 'Terrible' TB"

A woman and her daughter entered the waiting area of the TB section of Silverton clinic, Cape Town, and sat down next to me. I estimated the daughter to be in her late twenties. She wore a *salwar kameez*, somewhat ragged, the white material smudged brown with dirt. The mother was solid-set, in her late forties. They sat together chatting quietly, and then the younger woman acknowledged me with a greeting. Taking the opening, I explained my presence and asked them why they were in the clinic. They told me Liena (the younger woman) had "terrible" TB and the clinic knew her partner well for defaulting on his treatment. Tearfully, Liena explained to me that he refused treatment; that they slept in a bed together and he coughed on her; that he spat into a bucket next to the bed that she had to clean. He was also, she said, using "drugs." (I, not wanting to disrupt the flow of the narrative, did not ask for clarity on what drugs, but in all likelihood, this was methaqualone, as "drugs" was used synonymously with the local name, mandrax.) She and her mother could not, she could not, "take it anymore." They were therefore in the clinic to try to persuade the clinic staff to get her partner admitted to DP Marais. Having made this explanation, she turned to her mother and said to her, "We should also take the test while we are here. . . ."

Appeal 2: "He Is Spitting All Over the Yard!"

In December 2014, a year later, in the TB waiting room of a clinic in a different part of the city, I heard a story of striking similarly. A young mother sat breastfeeding a tiny baby, swaddled in a fuzzy pink blanket. Next to them sat an older woman, neat and scarfed, with a child of about a year old on her lap. There was an ease and warmth to the younger woman, so I approached and started to chat. How old was her baby? "Ten days," she replied. I asked if she was waiting for treatment and she explained that no, no, she (Daniyah) and her mother in law (Aafiyah, the woman sitting next to her) were there for the children's TB prophylactic treatment.[4]

Aafiyah took up the narrative. She explained that her ex-husband, the children's grandfather, was sick with TB and did not want to be on treatment. She said that though they had been divorced for seven years, he still lived in a shack in the yard and—as was common with yard dwellers—he still came into the house for food and to use the bathroom.[5] Their small house was full; in addition to Daniyah, Aafiya's two daughters, aged fifteen and seventeen, and her eldest son, aged thirty-three, were also in residence. And during the day, Aafiyah also cared for her grandchildren, Daniyah's children (the new baby and a four-year-old), the one-year-old on her lap, and another four-year-old. Her ex-husband's refusal to take medication rendered him continually infectious and all the children, including the newborn baby, were on prophylactic treatment.

Why, I asked, did Aafiyah's ex-husband not want to take his treatment? Aafiyah said she didn't know. I pressed the conversation into the area of my suspicions. Was he using any drugs, "buttons" (mandrax), perhaps? I asked, hesitantly. He was. A lot. And he drank alcohol, every day. Did he want to stop his substance use? I enquired. (At this point, I too had bought and was replaying the idea that successful TB treatment was impossible in the context of habitual substance use. This view I came to change, as will become apparent later.) His expressed wish, said Daniyah, was to "die in peace." "We want to send him away to somewhere like Brooklyn [Chest TB hospital] . . . but we don't know how."

As Daniyah was called away into the clinic room, Aafiyah continued explaining their plight. "He is spitting all over the yard! . . . I can't take it anymore! I'm tired. . . ." And, drawing on addiction language of being "clean" or not, she said, "He had MDR TB . . . they say he's clean from MDR TB, now he only has TB-TB." By TB-TB, she meant drug-sensitive TB.[6] She said that TB nurses frequently phoned the house seeking her ex-husband and trying to persuade him to come for treatment. She expressed frustration that he wanted a social grant, but since he did not meet eligibility criteria, he no longer wanted anything to do with the clinic. About this she explained, "He said they can't help me . . . I said, they won't help you because you are a druggie. . . ." And, in a lament, "He smokes [drugs] in the yard, there by my house. . . ." Finally, she told me that she had sought support from the police by requesting an interdict against her ex-husband, which would force him to stay out of the house. And, in a moment which truly signaled how stuck she was, said, "The magistrate told me if he hits me, I can use it [to put him in jail] . . . I don't know who to go to, if I can get a social worker, or. . . ."[7] She didn't finish her sentence.

In both these situations, two women, one older, one younger, were together in a TB clinic seeking protection through hospital sequestration for a male family and household member who was using substances, not taking TB treatment, and worryingly infectious. The appeals were well crafted, and I suspect that in both cases, I was engaged, at least partially, as a potentially useful ally, someone who would listen and who could perhaps be persuaded to use whatever influence I had to further their cause.

In telling me that her partner had a "terrible" case of the "bad" TB (MDR), Liena was indicating that she was in danger of something that was worth fearing. By telling me her partner refused treatment, that they slept in close confines, that he coughed "on" her, and that she was handling his sputum, she was further building a case for his bad behavior and her innocent vulnerability to infection. By adding that he used drugs, she was framing her partner's behavior as immoral and uncontrollable. The statement that "they couldn't take it anymore" added the indication that they had been long suffering without support. She was building herself a powerful case for state protection. And finally, by turning to her mother and saying they should take the test, she was presenting herself both as worried and as a responsible health-seeking citizen.[8]

Similarly, Aafiyah and Daniyah drew on the horror and risk of infectious sputum ("He is spitting all over the yard!") from an unapologetic drug user ("he smokes . . . there by my house"), whose self-interest was demonstrated by his refusal to take treatment unless it came with the benefits of a social grant. They too presented their own long-suffering status and the fact that their energies were depleted. Their story had two additional layers: there were children at risk and in need of protection, and the law could only protect them if they experienced the immediate tangibility of physical violence but could offer no protection from potential TB infection and the harms that that would inflict. Unable to mobilize legal protection, Aafiyah and Daniyah were protecting the children physiologically through prophylactic treatment and working on other options— and at the top of the list of options was hospitalization.

THE MAKING OF UNRULY PATIENTS

As I listened to these women I did not yet know how people who used drugs were set up by the health care system to be "unruly" (Versfeld et al. 2018; Scheibe et al. 2017; Versfeld et al. 2020). It was when I started working with people who used drugs through an advocacy and service provision nonprofit organization, TB HIV Care,[9] that I began to understand the ordeal of trying to access health care for people who used drugs. For anyone, a clinic visit frequently takes a whole morning and sometimes creeps into the afternoon. Patients must arrive early to be sure to be attended to that day (wait); the patient folder has to be made or found (wait); the counsellor or nurse needs to become available (wait); the doctor, if needed, needs to become available (wait); and medication needs to be doled out (wait). Even patients who are coming in for daily DOTS—a process of observation that does not require the rigmarole of a full clinic appointment—can wait—sometimes, though not generally—for more than an hour simply to have someone watch them swallow their tablets and provide the needed tick on their treatment cards. The requirement of supplication was often asserted through clinic staff simply not acknowledging a patient's presence until they were ready (and willing) to attend to them. Inadequate supplication could be punished by the withdrawal of caring care. "They *must* wait!" a nurse commented about patients who were grumbling at the slow service, "We are not a fish and chips shop!"

For many people who use substances, especially those living on the street, life is a treadmill of trying to generate enough income to afford the substance needed, getting to the place of drug sale (often a substantial walk from the place where income can be generated), using to stave off withdrawals, and starting again. For these people, time is a precious commodity that waiting eats up, while the fear of withdrawal, or withdrawal itself, sets in. For those who are intoxicated, a different challenge prevails—hiding their state, or risk a public scolding, or refusal of care. Being in health facilities at all, if identified as someone who used substances, often risked scolding or demeaning treatment. People who used drugs told me of having their test results relayed in public spaces and their right to privacy being completely disregarded by health care workers who lived in the same neighborhoods as them. They spoke about being told they were not worthy of treatment and at fault for all their own health woes. "Doing a thing" for their own health required, as one individual told me, accepting being "treated like dogs," and facing that, another explained, took "being nearly dead." It was not, of course, that every health care provider behaved like this or that such behavior was accepted in every facility. But stories of poor treatment have great currency as they circulate in networks of people who use drugs. Their power lies in the possibility of bad treatment they present. Facing that takes exceptional courage.

HOSPITAL POSITIONING

In February 2015, I conducted brief substance use screenings on as many of the patients in the Delft South TB clinic waiting room as I could, using a tool I had developed in partnership with DP Marais staff for in-hospital use.[10] The clinic served everyone in the immediate environment. My plan was to contrast the rates of substance use I found there with the levels of use I found in hospitalized patients (described in Chapter 4). Out of the 200 patients being treated in the clinic at that time, I screened sixty-three—these were the patients who were either early in their treatment stage (and therefore required to come in every day) and those who were coming for monthly check-ups. Of these, fifty-eight met my inclusion criteria (they were over eighteen years, their files were accessible, and they were currently on TB treatment). The results were telling. Despite the fact that Delft South is renowned for high levels of substance use, levels of drug use reported in the clinic were far lower than the DP Marais patient folder records suggested. Only 7 percent ($n = 4$) of the Delft South patients reported tik use at the time of becoming ill, and likewise, only 7 percent ($n = 4$) reported using mandrax at the time of becoming ill. No patients reported heroin use. A total of only 6.8 percent used one or more of tik, mandrax, and/or heroin at the time of becoming ill, as opposed to the 26.1 percent found in DP Marais. Though alcohol use comparisons were undermined by the measurement challenges in the hospital (outlined in Chapter 4), in terms of levels of people who use drugs, DP Marais was in a different league.

The high rates of people who use substances in the hospital, as presented in the previous chapter, are a consequence of the hospital's positioning within the broader system—as a place of care and containment of "unruly" patients—for families and household members, other health care workers, and sometimes patients themselves. The individual wants of a health care provider, family member, or patient were not meant to play into decisions about who was provided with a bed. Patients who were being referred on "medical grounds," meaning that they were simply too ill to be likely to be able to safely finish their treatment at home, were always meant to be first priority. DP Marais staff did try to privilege these patients by accepting referrals from tertiary hospitals—where patients were likely to be even sicker—over referrals from clinics.[11] The hospital chief executive officer frequently encouraged (or admonished) staff to be firmer in their stance toward patients referred on "social" grounds. But the hospital staff were well aware of the role they played in the larger scheme of health care provision and that, in accepting some referrals, they were serving families and their colleagues in clinics as much, if not more, than the patients themselves. While there were beds available in the hospital (which was not always the case), they did accept (and, as far as possible, keep) patients in the hospital where the dominant needs were "social" as opposed to "medical." Admissions were refused if the doctors suspected the patient was too ill for the medical resources the hospital had to offer, or—sometimes—if they assessed that the referral was made in order to "dump" a patient for whom no one else in the health care system wanted to take responsibility. Such latter refusals were, however, infrequent and often only after multiple attempts as the same patient revolved through facility options.

In setting up binary tropes of the "good" and "unruly" patient, I do not mean to imply their simplistic veracity or that patients were either neatly one or the other. A "good" patient might turn unruly, or an unruly patient might turn good. They could not, though, be both good and unruly at once, because the key characteristic of a good patient was consistency. One way in which unruly patients turned good was when a patient who was erratic on treatment requested his or her own hospital admission, which was not uncommon. On the same benches where I had first seen Bessie, I met a man of about fifty years of age. He was, he said, on his second "round" of TB treatment. He had started well on the last one but then started drinking too much and stopped taking his medication. Now he was worried that he would do the same again. And so he was in the clinic with a two-pronged quest. He was struggling with diarrhea and vomiting as negative side effects of his medication and he wanted help with this. And he was there to request admission into DP Marais for the rest of his treatment so he could be sure to complete it "properly." It was not unusual for patients—even those habitually using substances—to request admission to DP Marais themselves, especially when there were children in the house, and the TB-affected person was fearful that they would transmit the infection. As I turn to in Chapter 7, staying in DP Marais was sometimes framed as the best option by patients themselves. In the chapter that follows, however, I turn to all the systems of containment (which ranged from encouragement to coercion) the hospital team set in place for people who were less enthusiastic about their inpatient status than the staff thought they should be.

6 · CARE TO CURE

ARRIVAL

A stark white sign is stuck to the red brick wall next to the hospital gate, under circles of razor wire. It is crested with faded government logos and reads DP MARAIS HOSPITAL: TB IS CURABLE WHEN YOU COMPLETE YOUR TREATMENT.

How might we read this sign that greets, if not necessarily welcomes, patients and their visiting family members arriving at DP Marias? The message of hope ("TB *IS* CURABLE WHEN YOU COMPLETE YOUR TREATMENT") is one that health care providers frequently provide patients. But it could also be read as a message of individual responsibility: "TB IS CURABLE WHEN *YOU* COMPLETE YOUR TREATMENT." And for those arriving in the hospital after erratic treatment behavior—sometimes on, sometimes off—it could also be read as an admonishment: "TB IS CURABLE WHEN YOU *COMPLETE* YOUR TREATMENT."

The sign leaves out two additional phrases that would make it more accurate. The first, "if you have a strain susceptible to the medications available," recognizes the inadequacy of the treatment available (see Chapter 1) and the fact that some people will have a drug-resistant infection that does not fit into the category of treatable. Once a person with XDR TB has not been cured of TB after an extended period of hospitalized treatment (at least twelve months, but sometimes lasting up to two years), the person is discharged, despite still being infectious, with death the obvious long-term (or perhaps short-term) outcome. The potential consequences of this are dire: others may well suffer the same fate. When I spoke to health care providers about this, they expressed resignation with reaching the end of the line of the capacities of the system. What else, after all, can be done? But none of this information fits on a sign.

The second omitted clarification is "and you receive the right medication, in the right dosages." Standardized treatment does not always meet the dosage needs of TB patients, even in cases of drug-sensitive TB (Wilby, Ensom, and Marra 2014). While I was in the hospital, the doctors would measure the rifampicin levels of

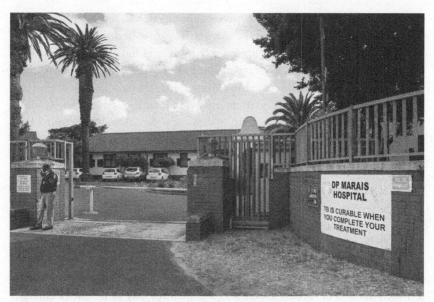

FIGURE 6.1 The entrance to DP Marais TB Hospital, Cape Town.

patients who were not making the expected recovery and would increase the pre-scribed dosages where levels were found to be subtherapeutic. But the generic care processes required in widespread public health initiatives do not allow for such individualized "tinkering" (Mol et al. 2010, 14)[1] and tuning of medication pro-vided. People who "failed" to heal were often assumed to be quiet "defaulters," especially if they were using recreational drugs. This was not just for TB. During my research, I was frequently asked by health care providers about people smoking ARVs for a "high." A widely quoted article indicated that pre-ART resistance had been found in some people initiating on ART. The authors argued that this was a consequence of ARV being sold by HIV patients who had been prescribed ART and being smoked as a cheap (illegitimate) high, resulting in missed doses for people making the sales and (potentially) pretreatment resistance for smokers (Grelotti et al. 2014).

What ensued was a media frenzy, which gave rise to public "knowledge" that smoking antiretrovirals was a common practice. This is disputed by people who use drugs—the buzz efavirenz might provide just is not worth the effort of smoking it—but it seems that no one bothered to ask them. What was happen-ing was more quotidian—changes in the genetic structure of the virus that were occurring with increasingly widespread treatment at expected rates (Manasa et al. 2012). The real explanation is not quite as titillating, though, and—even in health circles—the myth of the unappreciative patient benefiting from the needs of the bad drug user holds strong.

Generic systems of care cannot meet everyone's needs. Yet they are assumed to meet enough of the basics that the sick person can make do, if they really want to. In this chapter, I show how powerful narratives of individual responsibility worked alongside processes of responsibilization—the devolution of responsibility for health and wellness to the citizen, rather than the state—in the hospital.[2] These narratives were particularly evident in the "education" sessions provided to patients by the occupational therapy department. I examine how hospital staff tried to hold people in the hospital when they wanted discharge and show just how complex the dynamics can become as the needs of patients, their families and household members, and the broader community at risk of TB infection, come into tension with each other.

Anthropological work on institutional care has tended to focus on discrimination and violence "found at the very heart of compassion" (Ticktin 2006, 34) and on the systemic failures of institutional care (Biehl 2005; Gibson 2004; Garcia 2010; Street 2014), rather than on successful care provision. Exploring successful care provision is, as Todd Meyers (2013) has illustrated, complicated by the ways in which notions of success in care and therapeutics may be distinctly different between caregivers and patients.

In contrast, the anthropology of nurturing care has largely tended toward focusing on the intimate relations between individuals at the level of household and neighborhood relations (see, for example, Han 2011; Henderson 2011). Care tends to be presented as personally and effortfully provided on an intimate level in a lacuna of adequate state provision. Stressing that care must be understood as something that happens *between* people, Julie Livingston's (2012) work on a cancer hospital in Botswana provides one of the few examples in anthropology of the nurturing aspects of care that happen in an institution.

My own perspective is that the anthropological critiques of a thwarted, misguided, or insidious state (Mahon and Robinson 2011) carry the implicit reasoning that the state can and should provide care. Indeed, Foucault (2003) reminds us that the role of the state is not only that of control, surveillance, and discipline of the population but also includes care.[3] The critiques of state care that are provided only make sense against this reasoning. My ethical approach is to examine the dynamics of state care with an eye to assisting and strengthening "good" care. The question, of course, is what "good care" looks like. Annemarie Mol and colleagues define "good care" as "persistent tinkering in a world full of complex ambivalence and shifting tensions" (Mol et al. 2010, 14). This chapter shows how there were certainly substantial doses of "good care" at DP Marais. At the same time, the tensions between providing care and protection for individuals, families, other patients, staff, and the population at large while also honoring individual human rights (Harper 2010) were often apparent.

YOUR HEALTH, YOUR ILLNESS,
YOUR RESPONSIBILITY: THREE SITUATIONS

Situation 1: In "Class"

Twice daily, clearly and deliberately, Wendy would call individual group members over the hospital intercom system. While she never announced why the call was being made, it was common knowledge in the hospital what being called to the "group room" meant. Patients were referred to Wendy's session because they were deemed by hospital staff to either be a substance (ab)user or to be at high risk of becoming one. Attendance was not voluntary; staying in the hospital was often made contingent on going to "classes." The groups were run on AA principles. Overcoming denial, public acknowledgment, and acceptance of a "problem" were seen to be the first steps to tackling that problem, and publicly "outing" patients was part of the "name and shame" philosophy of the group. Abstinence was, at all times, the goal taught in these sessions. The mantras, "Just [stay abstinent] for today" and "No to the first one!" were inculcated as a means of building self-control. It was also understood that people who used substances did not "know themselves" or have a strong enough relationship with their "higher power." Reigniting a relationship was a key aim of the group sessions.

One day, a few weeks into an eight-week cycle, a group sat in its usual circle of chairs. Wendy was met with dubious expressions when she pulled out a handheld mirror and told group members that they would be getting to know themselves by facing themselves in the mirror. Each member would, she explained, come up to the mirror, look themselves in the eye, greet, and say, "I would like to get to know you. I love you. I forgive you for what you have done." She asked if anyone had done this before. There was the scratchy silence of no replies. Then Celeste ventured, "*Dis 'n bietjie scary!*" (That's a little scary!).

Jacob, early thirties, with a street-walk swagger, was the first to get up to stand in the center of the group. Peering into the mirror, he pretended to squeeze a pimple and greeted himself, with a lift of his chin, "*Awe my broe!*" (Hey brother!) Wendy's voice was tight with a reprimand as she told him to greet himself, not some other guy. Then she guided him as he haltingly made his way through the required statements of self-love and loathing. As he sat down, Jacob's expression turned inward, and he sank his head into his hands. One by one, each of the others in the room took their turn. Quiet tears appeared as they looked at and spoke to themselves.

In the discussion afterward, all expressed some sense of the profound, except for Timothy, an older man, who said he felt silly standing there, talking to himself. Wendy challenged him, saying that he needed to learn to face what was inside him, that they all needed to overcome the self-distancing that happens during substance (ab)use. (It's you, not the exercise, silly.) Jacob—all swagger deflated—started to cry as he spoke about how hard it is to face yourself, to get to know oneself again. Looking away when one passes or sees a reflective surface is, Wendy explained, characteristic of an addict—you no longer want to see yourself. What they needed to do, she explained, was to go through a process of uniting the two selves, though exactly what those two selves were was something she did not go into.

Situation 2: Puzzles down the Empty Passage

The room where the MDR patients had their occupational therapy sessions was down a quiet, locked passage separated from the rest of the hospital for reasons of infection control. The room was bare—windows without latches and linoleum tiles that flapped up on the floor, tripping shuffling feet. I arrived one day to find the group separated into two circles of chairs. Each group was given a mixed-up twelve-piece puzzle made of a photocopied picture colored by hand. The groups were set to compete—the first to complete the puzzle in the allotted time span would receive a prize. The hunched men tried to fit the pieces this way and that way, but when the timer went off a few minutes later, neither group had managed to complete the picture. Soraya then repeated the process, but this time the groups were given the full picture of the puzzle to copy. This time they succeeded—and herein, explained Soraya, was the lesson. To me, the exercise demonstrated the depressing long-term effects of the weak apartheid education system; the puzzle should have been manageable, with or without a picture to follow. But Soraya's message was different: trying to succeed at life without a plan was like trying to do a puzzle without an image to copy. She was, she said, aware that each of them had goals; she had spoken to them all individually, but dreams "don't just happen." They needed to realize that attaining goals was a matter of positive thinking and the right attitude. Only they could change themselves. One group member ventured an effort to explain the futility of the exercise. "Where I come from everyone is using drugs in the house, so if you argue with one, you might as well argue with everyone." Change, Soraya forged on, comes from within, and positive thinking requires being grateful. "We like to blame other people," but you must take responsibility for yourself.

Situation 3: Guilty in the Library

A third and final example drives home my illustration of the extent to which the individual was targeted as the locus of change. This comes from an education session run in the library, a room with a long couch lining one wall, and bookshelves with crumbling, moldy, smelly old hardbacks lining another. The patients, men with drug-sensitive TB, sat in a circle of chairs. The occupational therapy staff were joined that day by a representative of the Substance Abuse Office of the Department of Health who cofacilitated the session on the workings of TB. During the session, a question surfaced from one of the participants: "How can you avoid becoming sick with TB again?" The visitor answered, "One gets TB if your body is not strong enough to fight it. If you have good food (like you get here at the hospital, with lots of vegetables), if you exercise, if you don't do drugs and drink, if you take your vitamins, and if you are clean, you will not get TB again." "This is the way to keep the TB asleep," affirmed another staff member. "Don't do things that make your body weak!" added a third.

Through all of this, one confused patient kept chipping in with rote-learnt comments, such as, "You must take your medicine!" Another kept a rhythm to his interruption, "Yes, I like the things you are telling us, I like the things you are telling us!" Then the conversation turned to treatment interruption. If you default, said Soraya, you will "go down and die." She explained—using war imagery also often used in HIV counseling—that the TB medication makes the "TB germ put down the shield and the spear it otherwise carries, and get weak."

A patient, Roger, interjected. He said he had seen the doctor "chasing people away" (refusing to give them treatment) when they are not taking their tablets (as prescribed). He did not finish his thought, but the implication was clear: who is responsible, then? "We're trying to give you information so you can make the best choice," responded Soraya, saying that Doctor S (the doctor referred to) was "very passionate about his patients" and that he tried everything to make them better. The insinuation was that the patient being "chased" must have made a bad choice, resulting in the doctor's response. Soraya continued, "If you are not taking your pills, you are going to make other people [in the hospital] sick . . . it is better you go home, and die at home." Roger pressed on: "But what about the fact that you go home, and you infect your family. What is going to happen to that person's family?" "I like it when you ask these questions," responded Soraya, revealing the origins of the phrase used by the patient with the interruption tic. But then she said, "You're looking for someone to blame, but you were the one to not take your pills, so it will be your own fault . . . you will infect your whole family, but you will blame the doctor."

The message patients were being given in all of these sessions was clear: your health, and your illness, your responsibility. (TB is curable when YOU complete YOUR treatment.) There was no mention of the fact that infection requires exposure, that TB is rife in poorer communities in Cape Town, that crowded houses, taxis with closed windows, and *shebeens* (one of the only places of entertainment in informal settlements) are all sites of transmission. There was no discussion of the immune-sapping effects of manual labor, stress, and sleeplessness. There was no mention of how nutritious food requires shops that sell it and sufficient income to cover costs (both of which are in short supply in townships). The immense structural difficulties faced by poor people in crafting life were reduced to a self-help narrative: if you dream, and try and take responsibility, you can (re)make your life (never mind your circumstances).

It was not that the difficulties of life were unrecognized. Skills sessions were run precisely because there was recognition that life was hard, but efforts patients made to express their structural constraints, the complexity of their lives, or the fact that they were not the only players engaged in their health care processes were consistently looped back to individual responsibility. The none-too-subtle implication of this, of course, was that patients were to blame for their body's weakness, for becoming ill in the first place. This was a marketable idea, for it explained why they were ill, when others in similar socioeconomic circumstances were not. It was a message I found accepted even by the questioning patients, such as Roger. After the session where he had pressed for answers about the locus of responsibility and the role of the hospital in protecting families of infectious patients, I found him in the passage and asked him what he really thought. He replied that it was difficult to witness when people do not take their medication, because *Hulle gaan agteruit* (They get sicker), and then they get sent home, and at some point they end up coming back. I asked what he thought the hospital should do. To my surprised, he replied, "Doctor is right because he [the doctor] tries really hard to make the patients healthy, and then they refuse." The lessons had done their work.

THREATENED DISCHARGE

The threat of being discharged ("chased away") from the hospital that Roger was referring to was another powerful tool used to persuade fidelity to the hospital rules. It was wielded with particular effect with MDR patients. Sufficiently healthy, newly arrived, MDR TB patients were obliged to attend a meeting in which they were informed as to hospital rules and afforded the opportunity to ask questions and request assistance. These meetings were led by the MDR ward doctor, Dr S, and they were attended by the staff members the patients were most likely to see regularly: the occupational therapy team, including the substance (ab)use coordinator, the physiotherapist, one of the nursing sisters of the ward, and, for most of my DP Marais research period, myself. The meetings were much the same each week; there was a clear emphasis on the lay of the disciplinary land, as demonstrated in my notes from one of these sessions:

"If you don't take your medication for three days I will discharge you," says Dr S. "Or I will put you in isolation ward if you can't walk [to the clinic]. I am very strict . . . you *have* to take your medication." He lists the places pills must not go: down the toilet, out of the window, under the mattress. Occupational therapy, he says, is considered part of their treatment. They must attend the group sessions. He goes on to say that smoking cigarettes needs to be done outside, but if anyone smokes dagga they will be discharged. One man expresses surprise, "Yoh! Are you serious? People do that here, in a hospital?" Somehow his surprise doesn't ring true and Dr S is careful to choose his words so as not to confirm that people do smoke dagga in the hospital, while still being clear that he will discharge anyone who does so. Alcohol, he says, is also not allowed; drunkenness is grounds for dis-charge. He explains that after they have been in the hospital for two months, they can get weekend "passes" to go home. "But," he warns, "if you don't return by Monday afternoon I will discharge you."[4]

While each doctor added his or her own nuances to these rules, they gener-ally applied throughout the hospital. Refusal of medication, delayed return from weekend passes, and substance use on hospital premises were all grounds for discharge, as were aggression toward other patients or any of the staff, any sale of cigarettes, alcohol or drugs, theft, gang activity, or interaction between men and women, or any general sexual display (the latter particularly applied to women). On arrival, patients signed their acknowledgment of the requirements of their stay. A disciplinary discharge could happen immediately, without notice. For patients, it meant leaving without the considerable support usually provided to departing patients such as transport home, ensuring that government-supplied social assistance in the form of monthly grants were secured for eligible patients,[5] or finding accommodation in a shelter for people who had no home to return to.

In reality, disciplinary discharges loomed larger in threats than in action, with one or two per month occurring in a rotating patient group of up to 200 at any one time. The work of the threats was mostly in their potential, rather than actual, implementation. It was far more common for patients who were felt to be disruptive to the general equilibrium of the hospital to simply receive an earlier discharge than initially planned. For this, the patients would be told that they were being discharged with the weekly exit group, because they were ready to leave. This achieved the same ends (the patients would leave) without inciting tensions. It did not exacerbate conflict between the patient and the health care system, or the hospital and patients' families, when hospitalization had partly been at their appeal. When hospitalization was at the behest of family members, or other health care providers, rather than the patients themselves, however, threatening discharge was counterproductive. In those situations, a whole host of techniques were used to keep patients in the hospital.

PERSUADED STAY

The narrative in the hospital is that all patients are there by choice. "You can't force a patient to be here" was asserted on numerous occasions. However, the expected length of time a patient would stay in the hospital was set shortly after their arrival in one of the weekly planning meetings, without the patients present. Staff decided that some patients should stay hospitalized only until they had passed any immediate health risks. These were those deemed to have a "good support structure" (family and household members who could assist them with treat-ment) and adequate "social circumstances" (sufficient resources for nutritious food and stable accommodation), who were able to access clinics for their treatment, and who were not known to use substances. Others would likely have their planned hospital stay stretched close to the end of their treatment period. The long-stay candidates were those with "weak support structures" (few or no people living with them) and "poor social circumstances" (homelessness and/or abject poverty), those who were unable to access an outpatient clinic (either due to distance from their residence or mobility restrictions), and those who were seen as likely to interrupt or stop their treatment (such as patients who used substances).

Patients did not always agree to their planned length of stay. Nor did their behavior always align with the rules they had agreed to and signed (not infrequently with the X of illiteracy) on arrival. Yet leaving was not always straightforward or a given consequence of unruly behavior. When the hospital staff deemed that an extended stay was an important ingredient for TB cure, various techniques were employed to persuade an extended stay. Some were more general and gentler than others.

Method 1: Gated Community

The DP Marais grounds were enclosed by a chain-link fence. Within these boundaries, patients with drug-sensitive TB had relative freedom of movement, with some restrictions: patients were not meant to spend time in wards other than their own, and there was segregation of the sexes. The MDR ward, however, was segregated from the rest of the hospital by a metal gate, under camera surveillance, and opened through a button in the nurses' office. Due to infection control concerns, MDR patients were confined to this ward unless they had a permission pass to leave or were going to a group session in the specially designated room in the occupational therapy wing of the hospital. Anyone entering or leaving the hospital went out through one main door, past the security booth, to reach the hospital gate. This was monitored by security staff. In order to leave, patients needed to show their departure permission passes. Failing this, attempted departure could result in being physically apprehended.

Viewed this way, staying in the hospital was a little less voluntary. In truth, however, the fence that surrounded the hospital was not particularly sturdy; for the agile, it was easy to climb over or crawl under (I heard reports of patients making a quick visit to the local *shebeen*,[6] exploiting the holes and weak points). "Jumping" was not a physically challenging feat. Moreover, people coming and going frequently left both the main gate and the gate of the MDR ward open. The segregation from the world "outside" was more symbolic than physical.

Method 2: Delayed Discharge

The discharge date of each patient was discussed in the planning meetings but ultimately decided by each patient's doctor. In the week prior to discharge, departing patients would, one by one, attend a "discharge planning" meeting.

Here the patient would sit in front of a panel of health care providers. They would be asked about their home circumstances, their knowledge of their various drug regimens, and their forthcoming clinic dates. If they were living with HIV, they would be asked if they understood that their treatment was for life. If they were HIV negative, they would be asked how they planned to stay negative. "Condoms!" was the correct (responsibilized) reply. They would be asked which clinic they would be going to for medication, how they would get there, and when their next appointment was. Dr N, who ran these sessions, would ask about work and, if they had been employed, whether they needed assistance getting their sick pay or a letter explaining their absence. She would check that those eligible for a social grant had received assistance during their stay from the social workers to get one. She would explain to those who were receiving a temporary grant that it would only last for six months and, after that, they would need to find work again. If the hospital staff decided after the discharge meeting that an extended stay would be preferable, the departure date would simply be shifted into the future.

Danielle, a twenty-four-year-old woman, had been in the hospital for about two months when she went through this process but then did not leave. When I asked her what had stalled her departure, she replied that "they" (the hospital staff) had decided not to let her go. I asked her how she felt. Angry, she admitted, but then quickly countered this by saying it was better; this way she would be on treatment for four months before going home. That left only two months of having to go to the clinic to fetch her tablets. I asked her if she knew the reason for the discharge delay, and she explained it was because she had defaulted treatment twice before. She explained that this was because she had been "too busy" with her "own things . . . the drugs." She followed this explanation with a tentative statement, "But I don't want to do that again this time. . . ." In that hesitant sentence, and her statement that a longer hospitalization period was "better," she presented the desire for a different outcome and doubt that she would succeed in meeting that aim once discharged. She seemed both angry and relieved at the power exercised over her.[7]

Method 3: Deny Day and Weekend Passes

One afternoon, one of the senior nursing sisters came into Dr L's room with a question. A patient was requesting a day pass to go and buy food, but his discharge was set for the following week. She was unsure whether she should grant his request. It was not unusual for patients to be granted day passes after they had been in the hospital for some time and had "sputum converted."[8] These slips of paper—given at the discretion of the doctors and senior nurses—provided license for patients to come and go through the front gate. Dr L asked who was making the request and, on hearing the name, said, "Not a chance, he is a drug dealer and the likelihood is too big that he'll duck . . . and he is going next week anyway." A pass was one way of giving the hospital "the slip" (absconding), without having to "jump." Passes were therefore given far less readily to people who were not trusted to return. Patients reluctant to be in the hospital in the first place, or assumed to want a pass in order to access substances (which was not infrequent), were often denied passes, as occurred in this case.

Method 4: Monitored Excursions

Prior to her hospital admission, Inam, introduced in Chapter 5, had been living under a bridge. Despite this, unlike many patients who had lost their national identity documents (often when their residence burnt down or, for people who were homeless, when their bags were stolen), hers were safely stored in the home of an aunt. An identity document proves citizenship, and this is required to access a social grant. One of the (many) ways hospital staff took care of patients was to ensure that they accessed these grants while they were unable to work. This money would accrue while they were in the hospital, so that they had a little reserve on departure. Usually if a patient who was not desperately ill needed to fetch an important document from home, they would be sent with the hospital transport to make the collection themselves. However, Sarah, the social worker, was well aware that Inam was struggling with heroin withdrawals, and she feared that a day pass might result in a much longer absence or departure from the hospital altogether. The auxiliary social worker escorted Inam home for her ID retrieval. Monitoring tactics were also implemented via the family for substance users going on weekend passes. One of the social workers would make a contract with a family member, who would commit to ensuring the patient's return to hospital at the end of the weekend. Where trust was low, patients were only allowed home if there was someone who could be called to account if Monday arrived and the patient did not.

Method 5: Forcing a "Red Ticket"

From my room where I sat writing, I heard Dr L in the passage outside saying, "I'm still not prepared to let him go because he will just come back." A few minutes later, he came into my room to explain (and to let off a little steam). One of the patients in his charge wanted discharge, but Dr L had no faith that this man would complete his treatment as an outpatient. "The first thing he will do is default," said Dr L. "No . . . the first thing he will do is go get his substance of choice and then he will default!" The "coming back" he was referring to was the unwanted kind that marked a patient a "returner."

Dr L explained that he was, therefore, refusing to undertake discharge processes for the patient and rather forcing the patient to sign a "red ticket"—the hospital form indicating that the patient was leaving against medical advice or consent. On hearing this, the patient had confronted Dr L, "You can't keep me here!" to which Dr L reported responding, "You are right, but I'm *not* going to discharge you." In cases where a patient signed a red ticket, the doctors would provide the referral letter directly to the clinic, but the hospital would not provide the usual support for leaving, such as the provision of transport home or contacting the household to ensure they were prepared to take over the care of the patient. Through forcing a red ticket, Dr L explained, he was requiring the patient "to vote with his feet." This would leave a clear paper trail indicating that he, the doctor, had not condoned the departure. Red tickets were a way of making departure less comfortable (and perhaps less likely) for the patient.

Method 6: Dose Them Up

In one of our many conversations over coffee, Dr L said to me, "We're losing heroin users." I asked him what he meant by "losing," because it had two potential meanings: loss through death or through patients absconding. "Over the fence," he clarified. Dr L said that he had one patient on 30 mg of diazepam three times a day, "Massive doses!" He said the patient had come to him saying he was suffering terrible withdrawals and that he wanted methadone and that, in response, he had explained that the hospital was not permitted to provide it. Without methadone, the hospital had limited resources at its disposal to ease the symptoms of withdrawal. This was particularly difficult for heroin users. What they did have was the sedative diazepam (valium), which was provided in generous doses. Sedation was therefore used in order to keep withdrawing patients in treatment while also trying to keep them physically and psychologically comfortable.

Method 7: Do Not Delve Too Much

The ethical balance one plays as a researcher of illicit substance use is always delicate, never more so than when a deadly infectious disease raises the stakes. I suspected that Felicity, who featured in Chapter 3, was using tik in the hospital. When she went home on a weekend pass and did not return, I had a crisis of conscience. Had I reported on her, she would not have been allowed home on a weekend pass, I thought, and she would still have been on treatment. My crisis of conscience turned to wracking guilt when she eventually did return, immobile and unable to speak due to a right-side hemiplegia, the cause of which was unknown at the time. Had I said something, would the outcome—the newly twisted shape of her body and the rest of her life—have been different? My discussions with the doctors about this elicited a variety of responses. While one said that I should have said something (more guilt), other answers were, thankfully, less certain. One struck me as particularly telling: "Sometimes it is a blessing not to know about patient's drug use in the hospital, for if you know, you may feel you have to discharge them." This, then, was the least intrusive strategy for keeping patients in the hospital—do not delve too much, for the more you know, the more you may feel compelled to act.

The multiple techniques described above were employed to reduce the chances of a patient departing from the hospital before the medical staff deemed it appropriate, especially if the patient was not trusted to complete their medication on an outpatient basis. Decisions took into account not only the health of the patient and their home circumstances but also the risk their discharge would potentially place on others. If, for example, a patient had four young children at home and was still infectious, greater efforts would be made to retain them in treatment. If a patient was still infectious with a drug-resistant form of TB, efforts raised a notch still.

Zandile came to my attention when I heard a commotion one day outside the nurses' office of the MDR ward. An unhappy patient, famine-thin and unsteady on his feet, was standing outside Dr S's office. A nurse commented that he had been bedridden for weeks, too weak to walk. Zandile had mustered the strength in order to petition Dr S to allow him to stay in the open ward, rather than an isolation room. Dr S was firm and resolute. An apology—for what it was not immediately clear—would not suffice. Zandile would be moved to the isolation ward until he either started to take his tablets or "passed on." Zandile, energy depleted and shaky on his legs, was guided back to bed. I asked Dr S what was going on. "Come and look," he said to me, and showed me two polystyrene cups—one a full jumble of colorful tablets, the other half full. These tablets, he explained, were found in the bed, under the blankets and in Zandile's clothing. Zandile was too sick to be sent home and too infectious to stay in the open ward. A few days later, he died alone in a small isolation ward.

After Zandile's death, the occupational therapist wondered aloud whether they should have done anything differently. Dr S shrugged, saying, "Substance use guys are always manipulative." Zandile's moral claim to care was diminished not only by his ambivalent relationship to care (for whatever reason) but also by his substance use.

I do not know why Zandile had so carefully and surreptitiously avoided taking his medication; perhaps for reasons of his own, or depression, or other mental health reasons, life did not seem worth living. Perhaps the handfuls of tablets just proved beyond his daily swallowing capacity. Perhaps they just made him feel too ill. But as he lay dying, he was a man infectious with a disease that will kill at least half the people who become ill with it. His untreated illness therefore placed others (especially the nursing staff who were not protected through medication) at risk. Isolating him was necessary in order to contain nosocomial (in-hospital) spread. It also shielded other patients from watching his death and their own possible fate. Isolating him was a clear example of care provided, not for Zandile, but for the community of patients, hospital staff, and Zandile's family. The exact foci of care were not, then, always in immediate view.

ALLEGIANCES: FAMILY, HOSPITAL, PATIENT

Rosa's referral letter into the hospital read:

> Female. 31 years old. [HIV negative. Patient] has a drug abuse problem. If possible can you keep her until [treatment] is finished because her family wants her to stay until [treatment] is finished.

Rosa left the hospital five days later. A note in her file described the reasons for her departure: "[Social worker] phoned [patient's] maternal aunt. RE [patient] requests to be discharged. [Patient's] aunt wants her to stay in hospital, as there is no need for her to be at home. The children are in her care and even they [the children] said the patient must stay in hospital to get better. During weekend [the patient] sleeps outside with boyfriend and abuse[s] tik. Requested that the patient stays in DPM for a few more months. [Social worker] counselled the patient about the above and arranged for her to stay. Patient still feels that she wants to discharge."

When the individual counseling that the social worker undertook with Rosa proved insufficiently persuasive, the doctor in charge refused to support her discharge. But Rosa was determined to leave, and so she signed a "red ticket"—making her departure (and the health consequences thereof) her responsibility. Rosa's case hints of the complexity navigated by the hospital staff as they sought to balance the needs of the patient and others, including health care workers, family, and other household members, who had conflicting ideas about the role of hospitalization. The hospital staff recognized and responded to the broader care needs of families, which sometimes had them playing a fine balancing act. Nowhere was this better illustrated than through Imran and Marlow.

Imran was easy to notice. He was young—twenty-two years—and from his somewhat childlike manner, he could have been younger. He had a half smile that was quick to emerge, thick dark hair, and an overtly flattened philtrum, which suggested fetal alcohol syndrome (FAS).[9] Although he was thin, he was far from wasted, as so many patients were. In his early days in the hospital, he spent his time cruising around the long corridors—sometimes at speed—in a wheelchair. One could always tell where he was, for he whistled constantly, in fits and starts of tunes. When he got to an obstacle, such as a step down to outside areas or a door between a ward and the open passages, he would hop out of the wheelchair, maneuver it as required, sit back down, and continue on his way. The wheelchair belonged to the porter, and Imran was simply using it as a way of entertaining himself through the ponderous, monotonous days. Chatting to me became another form of entertainment.

Imran was in DP Marais, he told me, because he had TB for the fourth time. This was not improbable. I spoke to a number of people who had gone through the full rigors of treatment three, four, or five times, some even more.[10] Imran's susceptibility to TB would have been influenced by the fact that he had type II (insulin-dependent) diabetes, in a classic co-constitution, because diabetes lowers immune defenses and increases the likelihood of active TB disease. What was unclear to me (or perhaps simply unknown) was whether he had had three previous episodes or one continuous one, which had waxed and waned in symptoms. The latter was possible, if not probable, because Imran mentioned that he had not completed his treatment before. (TB is curable WHEN you complete your treatment.) As much as his TB seemed never to have been "cured," Imran's diabetes was not what could be described as "under control"; he said he had been admitted to one of the city's largest tertiary hospitals, Groote Schuur, in diabetic shock multiple times. The last time that he had been admitted for diabetes before coming to DP Marais, a chest X-ray had shown the (re)occurrence of pulmonary TB. He said he was not even aware that the TB was "back." Such interplay of diabetes and repetitive TB is a classic example of a disease syndemic. In Imran's case, however, it was interacting with a five-year history of what he called "heavy, heavy" tik use.

Imran knew that erratic medication meant that he would likely not heal from TB and possibly that he would develop a drug-resistant strain. He had, he said, asked to be transferred from Groote Schuur to DP Marais; he was seeking institutional care in order to stabilize his life to the extent that he could complete treatment. By his reckoning, this did not necessarily include substance use cessation. When I asked him what he had thought of the substance (ab)use groups he had been obliged to attend, he gave a little shake of the head, as though he was flicking off my question. He had been through so many programs before, much more intensive ones, he said. They hadn't worked, why should this one?

With time, Imran seemed to get bored with the wheelchair, but his passage roaming continued on foot and we would briefly chat as we passed each other now and then. Initially, these conversations felt comfortable and open. When I asked him about his constant movement, he replied, with a characteristically impish smile, "That's because I'm selling cigarettes." Selling (as opposed to just smoking) cigarettes was directly in contravention of the hospital rules, and I took the openness as a sign of trust. It was he who gathered a group of men for a focus group discussion on substance use. But with time, the congeniality withered. He was never unfriendly, but his enthusiasm to engage waned. The planned life history never materialized, for though he had agreed to it, he seemed reluctant and I did not press him. With time, rumors and whispers about his in-hospital activities increased. It was said that he was not just selling cigarettes. These rumors implicated another patient with whom he had become friends, Marlow.

Marlow was a "medically complex" patient. Standard TB treatment had not worked, nor had the regular adaptations made to treatment regimes, and there were no obvious answers as to why. Shortly after his arrival in the hospital, Marlow became one of the patients visited on the weekly specialist rounds. The sessions held the potential for answers and the alleviation of pain and discomfort,[11] and generally patients looked nervous but also pleased—or at least relieved—when the cavalcade of doctors arrived at their bedside. Marlow, however, appeared disgruntled. He endured the greeting with a nod of a response but kept eating his apple and staring out of the window at the passing urban life. In some ways, this was an understandable, almost dignified response, for in classic medical style, the discussion between the medical staff did not always seem to account for the patient's presence (or the presence of other patients within earshot). Marlow seemed to be treating the doctors the same way—as if they were there, but not there.

Marlow was in the ward under the charge of the young community service doctor, Dr M. She explained to those of us on the weekly rounds, and to some degree to the ward in general, that Marlow had recently been admitted to the hospital due to recurrent TB meningitis.[12] Dr A lit up in recognition, "Have you heard this story? Amazing!" he said to us (and to the neighboring patients). He explained that Marlow had had TB meningitis for three to four years. He had been consistently on treatment but just kept returning for care, with little alteration to his condition. Marlow continued staring out of the window.

Dr A turned to Marlow, "Have you been taking your treatment?" Marlow was not forthcoming. Dr M responded for him, "His mom says he definitely took it five days a week, though he missed sometimes on the weekends." Dr A turned his answer toward Marlow, "Okay, so that means you're not taking your treatment." Marlow's tone was petulant, "I *am* taking my treatment." Dr A, with frustration, responded, "You're not taking it! This is a serious infection, you can die from it!"[13] And, turning to Dr M, he asked, "Is his HIV controlled?" She replied that Marlow was undergoing second-line treatment[14] "and not responding very well. . . ." Dr A turned back to Marlow, "You're not taking your tablets!" Marlow countered Dr A's frustrated tone with testiness, "I *am* taking my ARVs." His omission of TB medication was a defense and admission wrapped into one short sentence.

This conversation left me uncomfortable. By saying "You're not taking your tablets," Dr A was not saying that five days a week was insufficient; he was accusing Marlow of lying. Dr A was saying that admission of some slippage in the daily routine was, in fact, a cover for irregular medicating in general. A month after this conversation, Marlow's viral load—the clearest indication of health improvement in response to regular HIV medication—had dipped right down and his TB symptoms had lessened. It became clear that he was not a case of someone who was simply pharmacologically resistant to the treatment, which would have been exceptional because his TB was the drug-sensitive kind, but that, when not in hospital, he had not been taking his treatment, or at least not with the regularity required to make it effective.

Both Marlow and Imran seemed ambivalent about receiving care. The nurses complained that Imran needed their attention and care, but he made it hard to give. He would not be in bed at night but would be sleeping so deeply in the mornings that they were unable to rouse him for his insulin injections. Other times, they simply could not find him for his insulin injections. He was given a warning for the cigarette sales but continued his business. He would insist that his sugar levels were low, but when they tested him, his levels were around twenty, "way, way high." "Sometimes," said Sister Jones, "you want to give up on patients like him . . . but ethics won't allow it." Imran and Marlow were described as churlish on receipt of acts of care. Both circulated through the hospital in defiance of hospital policy. Sometimes, Sister B said, you could see that he had a "dagga face." I pressed her for what a "dagga face" looked like. "Puffy," she said. He was reported by other staff to be returning from weekends (escorted by his mother) smelling of both alcohol and dagga.[15]

Concerns about their behavior, which did not fit the model of a "good patient," rose a notch when Imran and Marlow became, as Sister J described, "thick as glue." The staff started to read meaning into the patterns of their movements: they would alternate their weekend passes and frequently ask for day passes. Was this because they were alternating their drug-buying excursions? The questioning and concerns came to a head on a day when I was not in the hospital. An elderly man in Ward 2 had been experiencing an increase in epileptic fits. The reasons for this were not apparent to the staff, but another patient noticed that the fits came after the older man smoked dagga, which he purchased from Marlow. The concerned patient *piemped* (snitched) to the nursing staff in charge of Ward 2. They spoke to the social workers, who turned sleuths: they devised an elaborate system through which the reporter could identify the sellers without identifying himself. Marlow was pointed out. He and Imran—both under Dr M's care—were discharged that same day.

The next day, Dr M relayed the happenings to me. She had, she said, suspected that both Marlow and Imran were selling drugs and that they had been working together for some time. Due to this, she decided to discharge the pair simultaneously, even though only Marlow had been identified. She told me she had done this hesitantly. She had called them into her office and told them that she was discharging them on a suspicion. They did not dispute her half accusation but simply said they would go and pack their bags. Shortly afterward, they came and sat outside her closed office door waiting for referral letters. On the other side of the door, Dr M was taking an angry phone call from Imran's sister. How could she discharge him on a suspicion? Imran's sister shouted down the phone. Did she not know he had never completed his treatment before? Did she not know what she was doing to his health by discharging him?[16] Dr M had replied that he was healthy enough to be discharged and that it was time he started taking responsibility for his own health. As a doctor, she needed to take care of all the other patients in the hospital, too. As Dr M described this all to me, her shoulders sagged. She had so hoped, she said, that Marlow and Imran would dispute her accusation, that they would "put up a fight" so that she could find a kernel of reasonable doubt that she might be wrong, but they did not. I was reminded of the words I had heard her say before, about having to assert her medical authority to make decisions that were not biophysical in nature: "I was not trained to do this. . . ." A day later, Marlow's mother laid a complaint, too. Medical staff frequently sought to hold social distresses as they intertwined with medical distresses, stretching them well beyond the realm of bodies and diseases.

Neither Marlow nor Imran were acting as expected of them as patients. They were not asking for discharge, for that would have put them in conflict with their families, who wanted them in the hospital. Nor were they behaving as if they wanted to stay. They must have known that their behavior was setting them on a clear path to discharge. In fact, some time after this event, I realized that I had, in all likelihood (if unsuccessfully) been part of Imran's own "discharge planning."

It was a sunny day, less than a week before Imran and Marlow's discharge. I was sitting in the courtyard of Ward 2—the ward for older, fragile men—with Jayden, who had requested a conversation. Jayden was neither old nor sick enough to require constant medical attention, but he was openly gay. A hairdresser by trade, he always wore a large, sparkling faux diamond earing, a bright scarf wrapped around his head, and a blanket wrapped around his waist like a skirt. This rendered him exceedingly vulnerable to bullying and sexual violence. The hospital staff told me that they had hoped that placing him in a ward with older men, where he was under the watchful eye of nursing sisters, would afford him adequate protection. It did not.

Jayden and I sat in the Ward 2 courtyard, slightly removed from the other patients, in an effort to gain a modicum of privacy. I was focused on his narrative of abuse at the hands of other patients. Nevertheless, I could not help but notice Imran (who stayed in a different ward but, contrary to hospital rules, was visiting in Ward 2) standing up from one cluster of patients, crossing the courtyard (perhaps ten meters away directly in front of us), and quickly handing a small package to an elderly man. Without any perceptible conversation, he returned to where he had been sitting. I could not see the contents of the package, but it was such an overt enactment of a classic drug handover that I did not believe it was genuine. I read it, instead, as a performance: a handover of an innocuous package intended to test my response, my role in the hospital, and the reliability of my promises of confidentiality. Later, after their discharge, it occurred to me that the handover may have been genuine and, if it was, Imran was not goading me as a test. Rather, through an overt act of rule-breaking, he hoped I would report him. If this was the case, I had been set up to be a switch that flipped the wheels of the disciplinary discharge process into motion. Had I responded, the consequences would have been twofold. My research with patients who used substances, which was always fragile, would essentially have been shut down (a researcher of illicit substances cannot be seen to be a snitch) and Imran's discharge would have been achieved.

Why this carefully crafted performance of deviance? Marlow and Imran could simply have requested discharge. While both were medically well enough, there were two possible outcomes to this that may have been unfavorable to them. They could have requested discharge and received it. Or the doctors could have denied discharge, on the basis of family requests and concerns that they would not complete treatment at home, and forced them to sign a "red ticket." Either way, the responsibility for hospital departure would be theirs, and they would have returned home in conflict with their families. Being forced to leave on "suspicion," however, set the families and the hospital in conflict, deflecting blame toward the discharging doctor.

Unruly Patients and "Good Care"

In describing the dynamics between patients and providers, I have avoided using de Certeau's (1984) concept of strategies (as the methods of the powerful) and tactics (as the means of the weak) despite its obvious applicability. Health care providers (the perceptibly powerful) do seek to produce regularity and stability, and the methods of patients and their families could often be described as ruses or tricks that do not necessarily challenge but rather work within power systems. However, with the TB–substance use co-constitution, the locus of power that induces fear and puts pressure on people to act was not always clear. Power was concentrated in the policies of the state and the actors who enforce them who can, for example, decide when to discharge a patient from hospital. At the same time, TB–substance use co-constitution generates a feeling of being out of control in health care providers who cannot always maintain patients on treatment. Moreover, the individual, once contagious, is imbued with some of this power, for they, too, start to have access to the power to live and let live, or die and let die, something generally registered as the ambit of the state (Mbembe 2003).

These unclear power gradients play into relationships between health care providers who are, as the previous chapters have shown, under pressure to attain figures, patients, and families. In the hospital, relationships between substance-using patients and health care providers are often strained, particularly when patients are seen as unwilling to be abstinent, lacking in appreciation for the care provided, demanding of unwarranted attention, or disruptive in ways that contribute to health care providers' workload. Patient compliance—submission to the requirements and the rhythms of hospital life and treatment taking—is fostered through rules and, when these are broken, threats of discharge. This, however, is only something that works for patients who want to stay in the hospital. Where this is the case, hospitalization is seen as the most likely way in which a patient will complete treatment; hospital staff may employ a range of combinations of methods to retain the patient in treatment, from disallowing home visits to forcing red tickets for departure. These are overt acts of containment and control, the exercise of biomedical authority. I caution against an overly harsh reading of these actions. As Dr M said, "I was not trained to do this." Her comment suggests the improvisational quality of care efforts that are framed within biomedicine but respond to social complexities.

Moreover, decisions about admitting, retaining, or discharging patients were made with consideration for patient health, home situations, risk faced by their families and the broader community, and the stresses potentially placed on other health care providers seeking to maintain patients on treatment. Scheper-Hughes argued in relation to Cuba's HIV sanatoriums in the early 1990s that "[a] sanitorium is by nature a dual and contradictory institution, an odd blend of care and coercion. The sanitorium serves two masters, and the sanitorium physician is a kind of double agent. During an epidemic, the doctor always has two 'patients': the infected individual, who needs compassion and care, and the community, which must be protected" (1993, 48).

I have shown how, in the case of the TB–substance use co-constitution, health care becomes an ethical practice of moral and pragmatic choices that go beyond interpersonal relationships. Retention and expulsion from the hospital result from considerations not just of the person infected with TB but also their families and households, the broader community (even population) imagined to be at risk, and, importantly, other patients and staff in the institution. Noting this illustrates that care is not always directly between people and that—as we saw with Zandile's death—care and compassion may be folded into overt acts of control. Care providers were not only in medical and ethical relationships with the individuals in their physical care. They were also in ethical relationships with immediate family and household members and, more broadly, with imagined people of the general population. They therefore worked in present time with multiple "imagined futures" (Jain and Kaufman 2011). In the chapter that follows, I unsettle another dominant narrative—the inpatient TB hospital as the surviving, aged child of the sanatorium, as a secondary choice to the ideal of "in-community" care.

7 · CATCHING BREATH
The Hospital as Restricted Respite

To the medical profession and the sanatorium founders, the facilities were a gift to the tubercular. To many patients, however, they were more like prisons than hospitals, in which the prescience of death, not the promise of cure, was pervasive. Department of Health officials were earnest in their efforts to secure public good, but again, persons with tuberculosis found the policies too intrusive and often manipulated the system for their own ends.
—Sheila Rothman (1995, 252)

OUTSIDE YOU CAN LOSE YOURSELF

To get to the women's ward in DP Marais, one had to pass either through a court-yard or under a walkway that served as a passage. On a sunny day, knots of women would loll in the courtyard, spread out on the patch of grass, or propped up against the wall that caught the most sun. On my way past one day, I asked a small group of young women—all in their late teens and early twenties—what they were doing. "Just sitting," came the reply. Grabbing the opportunity for conversation, I asked what they thought of staying in the hospital. "It's nice," came a reply. 1 suspected that this pleasant, minimal answer was because patients who did not know me well had no reason to trust that I would not convey what they said to hospital staff, with possible negative repercussions. But the tone of our conversation was pleasant, so I pressed for more. "Surely, there must be something that they didn't like? There were so many rules. . . ." I was corrected. It was precisely the rules that made the hospital "nicer." "Outside," it was so crazy that you could lose yourself. The hospital provided time in which to find yourself again, to reset dreams and ambitions.

The women's answers did not align with my expectations. DP Marais provides excellent and attentive TB care and life's essential needs: treatment, food (of a pass-able standard and with daily meat and vegetables), and warm bed. But everyday life follows a set, mundane, rhythm of sleep, meals, and medication with little else to punctuate days. Family visits are infrequent (if ever, for many) and trips home unusual. There are abundant rules and privacy is lacking—private wards were reserved for the dying and those posing a risk to others. Patients must live with the sight, sounds, and odors of each other—something that often led to annoyance and frustration, even the occasional physical fights.

Elsewhere, hospitals are described as places of waiting. Writing about children's experiences of being hospitalized in the other TB hospital in Cape Town, Kate Abney links the extended processes of waiting in the hospital to a state of "continuous liminality" (2014, 170).[1] Alice Street (2014), exploring experience of hospitalization in Papua New Guinea, writes about the frustration of waiting, the anticipation of hospital departure, and fears of home and family ties fraying to a breaking point with an extended period away from home. I had assumed that in DP Marais, time would also be characterized by an uncomfortable waiting—for health, for freedom, for home.

In this chapter, I present a pastiche of case studies, letters from patients, and my own field notes to reflect the processes and ruptures of hospital departure, particularly for people who were homeless, using substances on hospital admission, or both. I show that hospitalization was often experienced as a welcome period of respite, and leaving was often faced with trepidation. The prison-speak that circulated the hospital of life "inside" and "outside"[2] did not necessarily indicate a desire for freedom "outside." For many, the hospital acted as a buffer, protecting them from tumultuous lives, at least for a period. Jonathan Stillo (2015) has documented how doctors in sanatoriums in Romania leverage TB treatment to provide basic social welfare, and Erin Koch (2016) has shown how social relationships mediated by TB care and treatment are often mobilized by both providers and patients for broader health-seeking goals. In this chapter, I show how hospital staff sought to maximize their protective role through providing assistance in accessing social grants, and ensuring home placement on departure, family counseling and meetings, and the substance (ab)use classes. Yet, the models used, specifically the emphasis on abstinence in classes, sometimes had the opposite effect to that intended. Rather than providing the tools for reduced use and treatment completion, the assumed binary between (ab)use and abstinence set conditions for failure.

PLANNING FOR DEPARTURE: SEEKING A HOME

Robin was folded into the back corner of the hospital minibus, wearing the thin blue mask that (at the time of fieldwork) marked him out as a TB patient. He was a tall, delicately built, older man, perhaps in his mid-sixties, but perhaps younger; the ravages of life and the effects of illness often made patients look older than they were.

Prior to hospital admission, he had been living on the porch of some relatives in a neighborhood close to the city center. He had a history of alcohol use. Now he was approaching the end of his treatment and he needed somewhere to go when he left the hospital. It was Sarah's work to organize this, and she was sitting in the front seat next to Jonathan, the hospital driver. I, wanting to understand the ways that the hospital team managed these "social" aspects of care, joined for the day's outing The minibus was otherwise empty. We were setting off to find relatives, hopeful that one would agree to take him in, though Jonathan had not seen them or made contact for six years.

As we started to drive, Sarah tried to buffer Robin against the disappointment she knew might follow. She counseled Robin that if they could not find a place with family members, she would find him a place at a home for the elderly. He was old enough and his pension could cover the costs. But she warned that getting a placement would take time and he would likely need to stay in a night shelter until a place became available.

We drove following a combination of disembodied, American-accented directions emanating from Sarah's phone and the embodied but equally clear directions from Robin. "Continue straight," said the woman's voice from the phone. "*Reg af!*" (Straight down!) said Robin. Some half an hour from the hospital, in a neighborhood of small and squat, but neat and fenced, brick houses, Robin told us to stop.

A young woman—perhaps in her late teens—was passing as we alighted. She was wearing a smudged purple tracksuit and her eyes widened as she saw us, "Hello *Papa!*" Her mouth was full of gaps and brown stumps of teeth. Ignoring her, Robin went straight up the short path to the front door of the small, cinder block house. The young woman followed us into the yard, greeting again, with emphasis, "*Hello Oupa!*"[3] He barely responded. "Is this your real grandfather?" Sarah asked because the use of these terms for grandfather ("*Papa*" and "*Oupa*") could denote respect, rather than a familial relationship. The young woman nodded and came to stand at the front door with us.

The door gave way to a solid, scarved, and stern-looking older woman. She commented that her spotlessly clean house was messy, indicating that we had caught her off guard and that arriving unannounced was not appreciated. Sarah introduced us and asked the relationship of the woman to Robin. She was, she said, his ex-wife's sister. Undaunted by the tenuous familial link, Sarah explained that we had come with a request for a place for Robin to stay when he left DP Marais after his full six months of TB treatment. The woman was clear: her home was not an option. Her son stayed in the house and could not have them both, nor could she ask her son to stay elsewhere. Sarah said she understood and asked about other family in the area. We were told that Robin's daughter was at the shop she ran at her mother's house; his sister still lived close by.

Robin's granddaughter indicated that she would show us where to go and climbed into the minibus with us. Still Robin barely noted her presence, though they now both provided directions. The young woman gave us family news: Robin's daughter, her mother, had remarried and (as was not uncommon) converted to Islam. We drove a block or two down, to a house of similar dimensions as the first. This one had a little shop attached.

Robin's fragile blue paper TB mask was now soggy with spit. Sarah and I, invested in finding him a home, were both worried about the fears the mask would generate. In line with the morning's rhythm of double messaging, we simultaneously suggested that he take it off. He was almost at the end of his treatment and no longer infectious, and the mask served no purpose other than to mark him as a TB patient.

Robin's daughter must have seen our arrival through the window, for she met us at the gate. Of solid proportions and dressed in long skirt, a loose gray top, and a black and white headscarf, she contrasted noticeably with her gaunt father in his worn, hanging attire and her dirty track-suited daughter. There was a toddler at her feet—a great-grandchild Robin had never met. Robin and his daughter greeted each other coolly. There was no evidence of a close familial link, nor indication that it had been six years since they had last seen each other. Rather, they seemed to be neighbors who saw each other occasionally and held no great affection for each other.

We stood awkwardly outside the garden gate. Sarah repeated her pitch, making the introductions and explaining why we were there. Then she launched into a direct request: "Is there not perhaps a place here?" Robin's daughter, Rabiah, was firm. It would not be possible; this was her mother's house. Sarah pressed, was there not, perhaps, space in Rabiah's house? That would require her husband's permission, said Rabiah, and—indicating that this was unlikely—she added that they were newly married and living in a one-bedroom house. Then, softening a little, she asked if Robin's TB was cured. But then her tone hardened again, as she complained that Robin did not keep in touch, news about him came through others, and she had not even known he was in the hospital. Sarah was not so easily thwarted. She asked for contact details, so that she could call once Rabiah had spoken to her husband. With reluctance and a request for time, Rabiah acceded. "How much time?" Sarah wanted to know. "Two days."

Back in the minibus, hope waning, we set off again, this time for Robin's sister's house. A few turns later, we stopped at a house with a bright, white wall. Robin went up the walkway and knocked on the door. The curtains were drawn and no one answered. Robin turned the door handle and went in. We followed him. In the bedroom to the left of the entry, an elderly woman sat in the bed, blankets pulled up to her chin. Here the familial relationship was undoubtable. Though she was as tiny as he was tall, they looked alike. She chatted to us—friendly enough—from her bed. Sarah again went through the process of explaining who we were, and why we were there, but this time she emphasized that Robin had a pension. He would be able to pay for accommodation. Robin explained to his sister that he had lost his place in the house in which he had been staying before hospitalization, when the occupants had changed. The new occupants had allowed him to stay on the *stoep* (veranda) and that was where he got ill. Sarah followed up by saying the hospital did not want to send him back onto the streets because he would get sick again. Face creased with concern, his sister agreed that staying on the street was not a good option. A moment of hope. But then she said that no, there was no place for him in her home. Her son, his wife, and their children all lived in the house. Sarah said she understood, but tactically seeking a change of heart, she turned to Robin and said, "We'll get you into a shelter if they have no space for you here." And then turning back to Robin's sister, "How many rooms do you have here?" Three. Sarah nodded: "Then perhaps you have space?" The sister got up out of bed to see us off, marking the end of the conversation. As he walked up the garden path, Robin said, "*Laat dit goed gaan hier by julle.*" ("I hope it goes well with you here.") I could find no trace of bitterness in his voice.

As we drove home, Robin once again folded into the back corner of the bus, now staring intently out of the window, expression inscrutable. Sarah turned back from the front seat and studied his face before staring through the front windscreen again. We drove in silence. After a while, Sarah told Robin that he must not take it too hard. He must be disappointed—she was disappointed too, but they had other options. They would get him into a shelter and find an old-age home for him.

Shelters in Cape Town were both in short supply and often difficult places to be, set up as dormitory-style as temporary waystations, rather than as places that could be called home. For the most part, they required a small daily fee and that inhabitants exited for a substantial portion of the day. There often was no safe place to store possessions and levels of substance use among other inhabitants were often high. Substance use and alienation from home and family often go hand in hand. This meant that people such as Robin often faced an additional dilemma: How would they manage substance use, or abstinence, on departure? I turn to this below.

ON THE CUSP OF DEPARTURE

Jacob, in his thirties and portlier than the average patient, was singing his way down the passage when we came across each other. I greeted him and teased that in the same way, I could always locate Imran[4] by his whistling and I knew where he, Jacob, was because of his singing. In response, Jacob announced that he would be leaving the next day.

When I asked him how he was feeling, a look of panic swept across his face. He was scared, he said, because of the "things" he had been doing. He did not know how he was going to stay away from the drugs, the tik. I was surprised by the revelation. Jacob had mockingly swaggered up to the mirror during an exercise in the substance (ab)use class, as I described in Chapter 6. He had not previously seemed interested in engaging with me and throughout his stay had maintained that he did not use drugs and only drank alcohol. Sensing a changed desire to communicate but unable to stop to chat with him, I offered him a notebook. He could write down anything he wanted me to know. The next day, one of the nurses brought it to me. Jacob had already left. There was a letter in the front, in rounded handwriting, with bubble dots on each "i":

> Wow! What can I say? I'm finally going home. My time at DP Marais hospital is over and I'm going to see my family at last after almost three months of my TB treatment. I came here to be cured of my TB because I couldn't take care of myself . . . I was using drugs before I came here, and that was my downfall, but when I came here, everything changed in my life. I decided to attend drugs and alcohol classes to see if I could get lost of my addiction. I learnt a lot, but . . . since I heard that I can go home I am scared for the things outside, especially the drugs. . . . Now the time is here for me to go home I get even more scared, because the cravings are coming back. I even dream about the drugs. I didn't take it seriously in the beginning, but now I am starting to worry.
>
> I feel like a wild animal that has been wounded and taken care of, and now I must go out in the wild on my own. I know I must be a man to face my obstacles, but who will encourage me? I am so confused in this whole thing, but I will try to do what Wendy always taught me, and that is to take it one step at a time, because I really want to be honest with the man in the mirror.
>
> —Jacob (The scared man)

The day before her hospital discharge, Tammy, angular and always little disheveled, noticed me taking notes in the women's ward nursing cubicle. She had studiously avoided me before, but now she approached and told me she would leaving the next day. Was she pleased, I asked. "Yes," she said, then, looking at her feet and scuffing one shoe against the other, she contradicted herself with a little shake of her head, "No." "Why not?" Then, looking up, directly at me, "I was doing a lot of drugs there . . . for nine years I was doing drugs." She came because she wanted to get away from "the drugs and all those things. . . ." It was her fourth episode of TB and her family—including her two children—were going to be disappointed to have her back before treatment completion. As with Jacob, I left her a notebook, suggesting she tell me whatever she felt needed telling, and leave it with a trusted staff member.

Tammy's letter started with a chirpy, "Hi Anna," but quickly took on a more somber tone, as she elaborated on much of what she had told me the day before:

> I am Tammy. I am 26 years old and I live in Hanover Park . . . I have been at DP Marais since 14/04/2014 until [today] 06/06/2014. This time is the fourth time I have had TB. I had it the first time when I was 17 years old. I can't remember how old I was when I had it in 2012, the second time. The third time was in 2013 and 2014 was the fourth time. I completed my treatment three times. This fourth

time I am still on treatment and I am only finishing on 5 August. I have two children. A son and a daughter. Kaylin is three years old. Today, Ethan turns eight . . . I have used drugs (tik) for nine years, through my pregnancies and through [all] my TB treatment. I have never really managed to stop. I made many people's hearts sore, especially because I stole my family's money, things, food and valuables, just to get my hands on drugs. I even went shoplifting and I stole my children's clothing to sell. I stole and ran away.

She also described the effects of her enrollment in the "classes":

I was in a group with Wendy for a month. We spoke about ourselves and what we use in our home environment. I really used a lot [of tik]. I went on Monday evenings to the AA meetings [in the hospital] . . . I learnt to say "no" to the drug that I use. To say "just one day at a time" and "just for now." To stay without it I need to have made the decision to change my thoughts. That's how I will change my life. I am going to clean out my cupboard in the places where it is dirty.

When we had spoken, I had asked Tammy why she thought she kept getting sick. Her explanation was that she smoked and shared a "lolly" (glass pipe used for smoking tik) with a friend who had MDR TB. The TB was on the lolly. As a biological explanation, this fell short. The TB strains were different (Tammy had drug-sensitive TB),[5] and sputum on a lolly would not be aerosolized, though certainly breathing the same air as her friend could have provided the conditions for infection. But these technicalities are not what matter here. Rather, what matters is the way that Tammy linked tik use to her repeated illness. Like Jacob, she was afraid of leaving the hospital.

The fear lay in maintaining abstinence. Wendy's teachings, her exercise about the "the man in the mirror," her frequently repeated mantras about "one day at a time," "just for now," and "cleaning out one's dirty cupboards" all made their way into the letters I received. The emphasis on abstinence was echoed in the occupational therapy educational and skills-building sessions and was supplemented by a warning at the final discharge-planning meeting. "What will happen if you put the drugs and the TB against each other?" Dr N would ask patients in their discharge-planning meeting. "The TB will win!"

Writing about addiction on the Rio Grande in New Mexico, Angela Garcia (2010) argues that the dominant narrative of the inevitability of drug use relapse preempts the way in which patients cycle in and out of a treatment clinic. An expectation of repeated failure becomes self-fulfilling. William Miller and colleagues (1996) have found that a belief in the disease model (and the need for abstinence) is a key predictor of relapse in people who use alcohol habitually. If one believes that one drink will inevitably lead to uncontrolled drinking, it certainly does. Like randomized controlled trials (see Chapter 4), there is an "anticipatory logic" here: expectations create results, which confirm expectations. Where substance use (as failure) and abstinence (as success) are pitted against each other in binaries, there is no real possibility of moderate or controlled substance use.

The binary presentation of health as abstinence or substance use as sickness (and potentially death) underscored the fear of departing patients. Coupled with this was the way in which failure was presented as waiting for them—"just one slip." Facing this fear (of death itself) was daunting, and writing to me was one way of sharing it.[6] Patients like Tammy and Jacob did not know how to continue their TB treatment if they restarted or increased their substance use after discharge in the best way to minimize harms. The binary also set the conditions for misinformation to thrive. I repeatedly heard it said, by patients and health care providers, that the reason that the use of substances and TB treatment could not be undertaken together was biochemical. Either the drugs would inhibit TB treatment function, or the illicit drugs and TB medication would interact to cause an "overdose." One person described how he would alternate days of tik use and TB treatment, so as to ensure that he did not "overdose," setting up the perfect conditions for the development of drug-resistant strains of TB.

This is not to say that abstinence should not be an ideal for optimal health. Rather, it is to point out the knowledge gaps and incorrect assumptions at play. We do not have information about the biochemical interactions of the drugs in question and TB medication. And there is no evidence that TB treatment cannot be achieved when substance use is continued. This feels counter to experience because "unruly" patients who use substances are both visible and problematic to the system. Far more discrete are those people using substances who manage to fulfill the role of "good patient" (see Chapter 5). In Chapter 3, I wrote about the way that the sample of people in drug treatment centers only included those who had not managed to stop their use alone, shaping a skewed understanding of the nature of addiction. Here I note that, similarly, the perception that drug use and TB treatment completion are mutually exclusive is constructed out of a skewed sample. Evidence to the contrary, as Tammy provided in her previous three treatment episodes, is hidden from view. The messaging in the hospital, based on insufficient evidence, therefore set up a barrier to TB treatment completion.[7]

HOPE FOR A DIFFERENT LIFE

Celeste was noticeable; tall, she walked to her full height. She was often carefully made up, hair styled, clothes from the hospital donation box color-matched. She liked sparkles and bright hues, and would greet the staff with a corresponding brightness. One of the nurses recalled her arrival: "Celeste had [heroin] withdrawals, she was sitting here outside, but she really looked like, you know . . .

mad. She really had that wild look. She was always looking for a *pakkie* (packet) [of cigarettes] to smoke. And I told her, no, man, don't do that . . . but you could see she was not *lekker* (well) . . . but eventually she got better, better, better. . . ." Celeste threw herself into all the events and activities provided by the Occupational Therapy Department, winning that year's "Miss DP" pageant—a pageant judged on carriage and modeling style, rather than on looks. By the end of her hospital stay, she was earning money from laundering clothing and was none too shy in telling other patients precisely what they should be doing. She became a beacon of hope for hospital staff, an illustration that people who used substances, particularly heroin, could make a dramatic turnaround.

As her treatment completion date drew closer, Celeste exhibited a heady combination of excitement, trepidation, and appreciation. Her excitement was that she would finally have freedom and be able to spend time with her husband and children. ("I've been locked away here for six months, with only one visit home.") I was not aware of her family ever visiting her in the hospital. Her trepidation was related to the fact that she was exiting to a night shelter—she did not want to go home to her mother-in-law's house, for fear she would return to heroin use with her husband. Her nerves at leaving were further exacerbated by the fact that when she entered DP Marais, her youngest child was only six months old. He had since been cared for by Celeste's sister, and, now a year old, he no longer recognized Celeste as a mother. She was uncertain whether to claim him back or leave him with her sister, who wanted to adopt him. Her appreciation was that the DP Marais team had nursed her back to health. This was demonstrated in a letter to the local press she crafted and shared with me.

> My name is Celeste Herman and I'm writing this letter from DP Marais TB Hospital in Retreat, where I am a patient. In April last year, my mom threw me out into the streets. I've been a heroin addict for a couple of years, and despite my fair share of rehab attempts, I had not ever managed to stay clean. Through my addiction I lost everything, even to care for my kids. On the street, I hardly ever worried about food or even my next bath. All I could think about was my next fix and when evening came, where I would sleep. Late November, having lived this life for seven months, I was diagnosed with TB. I was skinny and weak. The one side of my body was numb; I had to drag my one leg as it took me 40 minutes to the clinic for my daily medication. A healthy person would take fifteen minutes. At the [community] clinic, I inquired about a facility where I could get my treatment and food. To my surprise there was one, but with a very long waiting list. Fortunately, a bed became available within two weeks. I was conflicted and had my reservations as the TB treatment was for at least six months. My first few weeks were terrible, I became very sad, lonely, withdrawn. The hospital started to feel like a prison— my bed space like my jail cell.

As my recovery continued I realized that there is more to DP Marais than my confined space in the ward. DP Marais has a staff body, which includes social workers, counsellors, psychologists, audiologist, doctors, nurses, occupational therapists, and they are dedicated to each and every patient's health. At a time when I needed it most, they showed me warmth, love and care. The Occupational Therapy Department is extraordinary! They have an alcohol and drug abuse programme. It consists of two hourly sessions per day for four weeks, an amazing four weeks! Each ward has a timetable with daily activities such as arts and craft, gym, social group, support group, leisure recreational activities. Income generating projects allow healthier patients to earn some money. This was where I spend my special holidays. Even though I didn't have my children to celebrate with, DP ensured we get Christmas meals and gifts, Valentine gifts, even hot cross buns and Easter eggs over the Easter weekend.

Today, five and a half months later, I'm 20 kilograms heavier, more educated about TB and HIV, and I'm clean. The social worker has arranged a place for me to stay when I leave.

I brushed with death, but I escaped because TB is curable and there are institutions like DP Marais. I'm so grateful for being allowed to share six months of my life with people who have so much compassion and experience in this field. I write this letter as thank you to DP Marais and all their staff. I am privileged to have had the opportunity to be part of such an institution.

Celeste had been allowed to stay in the hospital until she was almost at the very end of her treatment period, because of concerns that she would return to heroin use and interrupt her TB treatment. She had been included in the substance (ab)use classes and was able to generate some income and savings through ironing. Sarah had worked hard to find a place in a night shelter, and to ensure that Celeste had a temporary disability grant to cover—at least initially—the costs of this accommodation. Despite all of this, when Celeste left, she said, "I feel like we're kicking her out into the street."

Celeste and I stayed in touch after she was dropped at a night shelter by the hospital bus. A few weeks later, our relationship ruptured over a substantial (acknowledged) theft from an organization with which I had set up voluntary work for her. The last time I saw her, her eyes were askew, her pupils pinpoint indicators of heroin use.[8] The letter she had written was never sent to the press.

Celeste's family lived in the same neighborhood as some of the nurses and, to much disappointment, word of her return to substance use quickly became public knowledge in the hospital. The hospital staff were deeply disappointed. We all put her "up here," said Sarah, holding her hand high up from the ground and indicating how far Celeste had had to fall in their estimation. "So, there is no hope . . . ," said the ward clerk. And one of the nurses, dropping her characteristically brusque tone, said, "I actually admired her so much. . . . Shame." It was only the substance (ab)use coordinator who mused that Celeste's sparkle in the hos‑ pital had been suspiciously bright, suggesting that she had switched her heroin use for more easily available, and less noticeable, tik while she was under DP Marais' watchful eyes. Hopes of a different life were hard to realize.

"I MISS THE HOSPITAL"

It took me some time to find Lucy-Jane's initial referral letter into DP Marais. Her patient folder was bulging with specialist reports and letters referring her from one hospital to the next. These records reflected eight months of investigations and deliberations undertaken by medical staff to work out the dynamics of the infections from which she was suffering from, and to work out how to treat these effectively. When I did find the referral and read, "Female, 34 years, HIV positive, no fixed address, convulsions, repeated urinary tract infection, suspected [dis‑ seminated] TB," I was surprised to find out just how sick she had been. By the time I met her, her health was stable. She was one of the women working in the laundry room and chattily walking round the hospital. My field notes docu‑ mented her departure process:

> Lucy-Jane has been looking for the ward clerk. She needs to leave today—a couple of days sooner than expected—because she has found a job and the people she is going to work for need her to start immediately. Her discharge plan‑ ning was undertaken a few weeks ago, but departure has been delayed in order to allow her to go to Groote Schuur for a check-up, and because her disability grant, set up by the social workers, has not yet come through. Dr N, her ward doctor, is away, but Dr L and the pharmacist get busy with arrangements so that she can leave today. They bustle through arrangements so that she is in time to leave with hospital-provided transport, checking that her documents are complete, that she has no follow-up appointments pending, and that she has the necessary medi‑ cation and referral letter.
>
> Lucy-Jane comes into my office to tell me that she is leaving. Everything is organized. She says that she must stay healthy, because so many people here have struggled to get her healthy. "I'm going to miss this place," she says, in her quiet way. She asks for my number, so she can tell me how she is doing.
> —Field notes, 4 April 2014

One morning, a few months later, I missed a call on my phone from Lucy- Jane. Once home, I returned it. I asked her how she was. "Fine," she replied, but said that she was looking for new work because her current job paid too little. I told her that Dr N had asked me to pass on the message that the hospital was still trying to secure her a disability grant. Dr N also, I said, asked me to check if she was still taking her treatment. She was. Getting the dates wrong I asked,

"Will you take [your TB treatment] until August?" "Dr N said I must take it until December . . ." corrected Lucy-Jane, adding, "Please tell them at the hospital that I am fine." She said she wanted to visit, would visit soon, but she was struggling with money. It had been her son's birthday the previous week, and she had used all her money to pay for a celebration. Her hunt for a new job was due to the dismal amount her current job—the one she had left the hospital for—paid. She named the amount: R300 ($30) per month. "Is that even legal?" I spluttered the question, shocked and knowing full well that it was not.[9] Ever even-toned and tempered, Lucy-Jane replied softly, "I know it isn't, but I have no choice. I have nothing else . . . I miss the hospital. . . ." How many days a week did she work? Every day from the early morning, when she dressed the child and prepared her for the school day until late at night when she put her to bed. During school hours, she did housework. My dismay spluttered into the phone again, but Lucy-Jane remained measured, repeating that she had no option, she had no other home to go to.

Lucy-Jane, of no fixed abode before hospitalization, had hastily left the hospital (before she was required to) because an exploitative job offered her a roof over her head. The domestic servitude she described is common, though exactly how common is not well recorded. Poverty, inequality, and high unemployment create extreme vulnerability in young women from rural areas (Human Sciences Research Council of South Africa 2010). A history of widely accepted domestic labor exploitation (Cock 1989) means that employers can too often continue without raising attention.

Jane had originally come to Cape Town from a town in the Northern Province, a region known for flows of young women coming to Cape Town seeking a better life and finding themselves locked into exactly the kind of work Lucy-Jane was describing finding herself in after leaving the hospital. From what she told me, I suspect she had been previously acquainted with the conditions she was now experiencing. The irony of this departure was that in order not to lose this job, Lucy-Jane left the hospital before her disability grant had come through. Had she stayed long enough to get it, she would have had an income over four times more than she was getting from work, though it would not have covered the costs of her rent.

TAKING FREEDOM, GIVING TIME

In the previous chapter, I discussed the complex system of persuasive techniques employed to keep unruly patients—of all forms of TB—hospitalized, while also showing that hospitalization was ultimately an "opt-in" option for patients. I have shown how the prison-speak of life inside and life outside reflected people's feelings of being confined, rather than the reality of imprisonment. Hospitalization is sometimes medically necessary; it can also be socially desirable, especially

when life "outside" is very cruel. Time in the hospital was not necessarily characterized by supplication and waiting; it was also something to "sit in," to inhabit,
to use—a moment of respite, a place to catch breath, where people are buffered
from the cruelties of life on the margins. This chapter has shown that there were
reasons to fear discharge, especially for people who, like Lucy-Jane, Celeste, and
Robin, were homeless and those who, like all of those presented in this chapter,
were using substances at the time of becoming ill.

Recognizing the broader role of hospital time, staff stretched admission periods to keep patients with fraught lives in the hospital until the end—or very near
to the end—of their treatment period. This was despite the pressure on hospital
beds, and in defiance of management's requirements. "The one thing we can give
them is time," said Dr L. In the time "given," hospital staff sought to instill skills
and practices that would make life "outside" more feasible. This included the
"life skills" sessions described in the previous chapter. It also included the substance (ab)use classes. Staff also tried to ensure that patients were afforded the
state care they were due. Many patients arrived without identity documents and
were ineligible for social grants. Social workers ensured that by the time they left,
these were in place. For patients who had been employed, employers were con-
tacted, due sick leave was negotiated and (if possible) a return to work was
arranged. Where family relations were fraught, family meetings were called.

There is a long-standing debate about the role of hospitalization in TB treatment. As Paul Farmer and Edward Nardell point out, "In decades past, the argument was often between reformers and segregators: those calling for improved
housing and nutrition for the poor and those favoring removal of the afflicted to
sanatoriums" (1998, 1014). The emergence of drug-resistant TB provided new
charge to these debates. Sequestration of those who are infectious becomes
more palatable as effects of infection become harsher. But ultimately, in South
Africa, "in-community" care has won out, on the basis of human rights (L. London
2009), effectiveness and reach (Heller et al. 2010), and cost (Schnippel et al.
2013). This chapter has shown that hospitalization may be both desirable (a place
of respite) and undesirable (prison-like), which pushes us into rethinking power
and agency in relation to hospitalized sequestration. The cycling of patients
through the hospital was not only about a patient's failure to "get well"; it was—
as has also been discussed in Chapter 4—about the success of individual patients
in accessing state-provided respite when this was felt necessary. The question is
not whether hospitalization is ever appropriate, but rather when it is appropriate
and what is needed to maximize the positive role it plays in patients' lives.

In DP Marais, all the processes I describe in this chapter were designed to
lessen fear of departure. One hospital effort, however, seems to have served
to increase the fear of departure, at least among some patients. The approach of
teaching that substance use and TB treatment were necessarily oppositional may
have helped some patients to stay abstinent in the long run. However, the more

common and expected outcome was a return to substance use. Certainly, patients who were leaving emphasized the perception that abstinence was essential. This generated disquiet in those who were unsure that they would be able to do so. Critically, pitting substance use and TB against each other did not allow for the hospital team to work with patients to generate the knowledge and competencies needed to complete their TB treatment in the event of substance use. Time in the hospital, as a moment of respite and reflection, could have been far better put to use if the hospital staff approached it as an opportunity to work with patients to develop pragmatic ways of completing TB treatment, if necessary, even if using substances. I turn to discussing the shift to this latter approach in the concluding chapter.

8 · ANTHROPOLOGY
IN ACTION

"Brian is HIV positive and was diagnosed with MDR last year, and," says Dr S, "we fixed that, but we didn't fix his alcohol problem."

—Field notes, DP Marais, May 2014

It is completely different in hospital because it shelters them from everything until they go back onto the streets or back into their living circumstances ... we try and bring it all together ... but it doesn't work. Our patients go out healthy, and then they just come back to us. They are recycled.... [The chances of stopping drugs and completing treatment] is like a lotto for some patients ... what are the chances of some of them winning?

—Interview, Sr S, DP Marais, September 2013

RETURNING TO RETURNERS

Jeffrey, lying in the sun in the opening of this book, knew that he had impeccably played the part expected of him: he had avoided health care until he was too sick to make the choice himself, gained relative health under the watchful ("sheltering") eye of hospital staff, and had been discharged into family care. Then he ceased to take his medication regularly, left his parents' home, returned to living on the street and using substances, and developed MDR TB. What he did not know at the time was that he would also change the story. The next time he left the hospital, he completed his treatment, established a business, and remarried.[1] Had Jeffrey won the lotto? I don't believe so. Rather, as I show here, he demonstrates that when we look a little deeper, all was not as it seemed with the patterns of the TB–substance use co-constitution.

My examination of the TB–substance use co-constitution in this book has been guided by an underlying concern: how do we generate adequate intellectual and practical responsiveness to this specific co-constitution and co-constitutions in general? In attempting to answer this question, I have drawn on foundational anthropological work that has illustrated the ways in which conditions of marginalization generate health conditions, encourage substance use (often, but not always regarded as a health condition), and foster interacting health conditions, whether these are understood as comorbidities or syndemics.

I have, however, broken ranks in that I have argued that the continued foregrounding of disease undermines the power of ethnography to provide a rounded picture. Through examining the ways in which TB and substance use are understood and responded to, I have illustrated that illness and outcomes can be powerfully determined by the ways in which moral valences, explanatory tropes, institutional norms, diseases, and social circumstances intersect. In these configurations and interactions, diseases are not necessarily the most important players. As long as we, as anthropologists, continue to create an implicit hierarchy in which we privilege that which is classifiable as disease, we undermine our own efforts at drawing (and paying) attention to other, potentially equally, if not more important health forces.

Like others (Weaver and Mendenhall 2014; Engelmann and Kehr 2015), I have illustrated that co-constitutions form more than the sum of their parts. What manifests therefore overspills the capacities and the mandates of the policies and institutions designed to deal with the singular constituents. Public health approaches that respond to health conditions or impactors as separate forces will, therefore, not generate adequate responses to co-constitutions. Additionally, I have shown how in the TB–substance use co-constitution, symptoms and signs of illness and health become masked as these health forces overlay each other. This makes it extremely difficult, if not impossible, for those affected and health care providers alike to interpret the constitution of poor health and to respond accordingly. In this obfuscation, social relations come to play a particularly important role in shaping causal explanations and responses. This means that with co-constitutions, it is important to understand the cultural, moral, and intellectual frameworks at play, for these determine who is seen to be deserving, where blame is apportioned, and how the state inserts itself into the lives of individuals. In the case of infectious disease—where fear is exacerbated and the state has a heightened obligation to respond effectively—this is of magnified importance.

In this final chapter, I pull together an argument that has been building through this book. The problems experienced in providing successful care for people who used substances were perceived and described as a consequence of drug use. This is an oversimplification that elided the ways that sticky moral opinions, policy, and health provision processes set up people who used drugs with TB to fail. I further present shifts that occurred in DP Marais when attention started to turn toward the ways that health care providers were complicit in causing the problems (substance use and TB treatment interruption and/or cessation) they were hoping to cure. I outline key changes in the approach the hospital staff took. Through this, I show that moral opinion may be sticky, but it is not immovable.

REIMAGINING THE PROBLEM

It was not only Jeffrey who had diverted from expectations by ceasing to be a "returner." Lucinda (presented in Chapter 3) and Tammy (see Chapter 7) both told me how they had previously completed TB treatment while using substances. And my Delft South clinic showed that 37.7 percent of people reported that they had stopped substance use of their own accord when they became sick with TB, and 24.4 percent indicated that they continued using substances to some extent through their treatment. Acts such as these, which defied expectation, often went unnoticed. Those who left the hospital went unnoticed unless they returned again, sick, and there was ample reason for people using substances to do their utmost to hide their use from health care providers. Not only was substance use criminalized, but it marked one out as "immoral," "irresponsible," "lacking in willpower," or—at best—"sick" with another disease in addition to TB (see Chapter 3). It also increased the likelihood of experiencing stigma, poor treatment, or—in the extreme—exclusion from care (see Chapter 5). There are ample reasons for enacting the "good patient" and people who use substances and do so successfully go unnoticed. It is failure and challenge that is grippingly visible.

In raising the point that there are people (how many, we do not know) who quietly continue their substance use through the course of their successful TB treatment, I am not denying that—to some extent—substance use, by its very nature, complicates treatment. It adds an extra moving part to an already complex process. There is not enough information available on potentially negative inter-actions with medications, and health care providers necessarily err on the side of caution.[2] Moreover, as I show in Chapter 3, substance use can mask the symp-toms of TB and result in a reading of the body that misses TB or illness in general. And, as others have also shown (Knight 2015; Bourgois and Schonberg 2009; Bourgois 1995; Garcia 2008), habitual substance use is often part and parcel of life at the very margins, where the stability that supports TB treatment completion is tenuous at the best of times.

Health care providers, people affected by TB, and their families, held a com-mon narrative: it was substance use per se that shaped the ways in which people who used substance engaged, or did not engage, with the health care system. This aligned with their experiences. Hospital staff noted with frustration that the same patients who used drugs reappeared for treatment time and again, with diminishing chances of treatment success. In clinics, health care providers expe-rienced people who used drugs as erratic and difficult to provide care for, as undermining of efforts to attain the treatment targets by which their work was assessed. Family members who engaged with the health care system spoke of strains in the home, their worries that their family members would not heal, and their fears of infection spread. This narrative is also reinforced generally by most of the available literature and data, mine included, which suggests that substance use disrupts treatment. At the same time, my data also point to something else going on.

My contention is that the assumption that the problem of "unruly patients" was a result of substance use per se was generated through very powerful tropes about substance use. The moral model of understanding substance use—which frames use as a consequence of moral turpitude and lassitude—and the disease model—which frames addiction as a chronic, compulsive disease of the brain— are powerful explanatory tropes at play in South Africa, not least in the health care system. People who used substances were perceived as lazy ("They don't do a thing for their own health!") and at the mercy of their circumstances and addiction ("It's like a lotto . . .").

These tropes were evident in the way policy was constructed (see Chapter 2). They were also at play in the ways that health care providers in the hospital responded to people who used substances. In education sessions, TB infection and disease was explained in terms of pathogen, behavior, and risk while failing to acknowledge the structural violence that hewed into lives. Taking TB treat- ment (much like not using substances) was described as a matter of commit- ment, diligence, and willpower. Health care providers sought to create "good patients" through instilling fear ("You will die!"), frightening them into absti- nence ("The drugs will win!"), inspiring acknowledgment of individual respon- sibility ("You're looking for someone to blame"), and generating guilt ("You will infect your whole family"). Where patients raised the impossibility of their cir- cumstances ("Where I come from everyone is using drugs in the house, so if you argue with one, you might as well argue with everyone"), these were perhaps lightly acknowledged but generally brushed aside. These responses failed to acknowledge, as Paul Farmer (1997) pointed out decades ago, that those most likely to complete TB treatment are those most *able* to do so.

At the same time, health care providers were painfully aware that they were working against the contexts in which patients lived and that they had limited tools and training at their disposal ("I was not trained to do this"). Hospital staff, therefore, sought to provide a range of interventions in order to buffer patients from the stark difficulties of lives on the margins. These included coun- seling with patients and their families, assistance in accessing appropriate social grants, ensuring patients had a place to go to on their discharge, and—where possible—keeping patients in the hospital for extended periods if this was con- sidered likely to increase their chances of treatment completion. These efforts were made within the recognition that this would never be enough. As one nurse lamented, "You know that when a patient leaves here, that's it, 99 percent go back to the same circumstances. There's nothing in the community that will . . . it's not enough. And when you are hungry, and when you are poor and when you struggle you go back to what you have done before, and then it is just a vicious cycle."

In the face of the sense of futility this could inspire, responses to the immediate, legible, "medical" concerns, were, as Dr L described it, "a refuge." In all of this, substance use was being pitted against TB, and the work of the hospital was being pitted against the unravelling caused by the world "outside." A better approach was needed, one that generated less of a sense of futility.

PUTTING ANTHROPOLOGY INTO ACTION

In my first week of fieldwork, I was witness to the tensions about which substance use assessment tool should be used in the hospital. At the time, two tools were widely used in public health settings in the Western Cape. The CAGE tool is a short, blunt instrument, consisting of four questions, designed to test whether drinking is "risky," based on social condemnation (see Chapter 3). The Alcohol, Smoking and Substance Involvement Screening Test (ASSIST) questionnaire is a longer, more detailed tool developed by the WHO. This is designed to assess whether the interviewee is currently dependent on substances or future dependence is likely. The tool is also designed to be implemented as a "brief intervention".

For patients using substances, it can take up to forty-five minutes (if not longer), and it requires a certain level of motivational interviewing skill. Starting the conversation in one of the MDR TB patient intake meetings, Soraya stated, "We have decided to use the CAGE." Nora (the psychologist) tensed up visibly, as she made her objection. She was working in two hospitals and only in DP Marais one day a week, and she needed clarity that the CAGE assessment did not provide. Unmoved, Soraya made her countercase: her team had a high caseload, and undertaking the ASSIST was too difficult under the circumstances. Frustrated, Nora reiterated that CAGE, with its binary options of "high risk or nothing," was useless. The tension grew until Dr S lost his patience, broke his silence, and ended the debate: "You can't do an ASSIST assessment on my patients. My ward is a madhouse! The nurses are always busy, a patient died this morning. . . . There is always something going on. Under the circumstances, we *will* do CAGE."

After a few months of ethnographic research, it became evident that neither of the debated tools provided the information needed in the hospital. Assessment of substance use was needed for the sake of medical intervention and assisting patients to complete their TB treatment. What they needed to know was what substances a patient used, whether this use had been continued or stopped in illness and treatment, whether a patient was experiencing withdrawals (and was therefore likely to abscond if they did not receive assistance), and whether substance use had affected treatment adherence. The tools in circulation provided information on what substances were used and how much but did not touch on the other areas. Along with the staff team, I developed a tool that assessed whether substances were being used in a way that was actually (or potentially) disrupting TB treatment. This was the beginning of a process of working with hospital staff to distinguish between the purpose of their work and moral perspectives on substance use. This required reimagining the problem they thought they were facing.

CHANGE REQUIREMENTS

Throughout the research, I maintained discussion with a representative from the Department of Social Development. In late 2014, this representative presented some of the results of my folder review (see Chapter 4) in a provincial forum. These showed the high proportion of people in DP Marais who were using substances when they became sick with TB. It was clear that managing substance use in the hospital needed a thought-through response. Suddenly, I found myself working in a team—with hospital staff; a local nonprofit organization, TB HIV Care; and representatives of the Provincial Departments of Health and Social Development—focused on the development of a better way of working with the TB–substance use co-constitution in the hospital. TB HIV Care was a health implementation and advocacy organization working across the country. They gave a name and theory to the method we had come to through pragmatism in DP Marais: harm reduction.[3] Our approach did not include classic elements of a harm reduction approach, such as opioid substitution therapy (not legally available to the hospital), safe use spaces (a step too far for comfort), or needle exchange for people who injected drugs (of whom there were very few in the hospital), but our approach did share the central tenet of meeting the patient "where they are at" (Marlatt 1996).

For the most part, though, it focused on debunking myths about the TB–substance use co-constitution and working with patients to develop strategies for completing their TB treatment no matter what their substance use patterns or habits were. Implementing this in the hospital took concerted efforts to shift mind-sets of health care providers and patients alike. The overarching idea was that substance use and successful TB treatment were necessarily impossible partners. This was underwritten by the misconception that substance use would prevent the TB treatment from working pharmacologically, that concurrent substance use and TB treatment would result in "overdose," and that substance use inevitably structured life in ways that made regular treatment taking, and being "good patients," impossible. (The latter, of course, does not recognize the fact that drug users are extremely good at imbibing substances when the motivation is sufficient.)

WHAT MAKES A CHANGE?

In mid-2015, I organized a seminar that brought together practitioners, government representatives, and academics to talk through research and practice relating to the TB–substance use co-constitution. For this, I asked Soraya to talk about the "DP Marais Harm Reduction Program." A few days before the presentation,

Soraya sent me her draft talk. It was a description of the intervention program that was crackling dry. Knowing that despite the fact that she was implementing the program, she was suffused in doubt about it, I wrote back, asking her if she could try to talk about why "harm reduction is so hard to swallow."

On the day of the seminar, Soraya spoke bravely and eloquently about frustration, misgiving, change, and hope. She explained how she had started at DP Marais eight years before and how she had been mentored in her approach to substance use by Wendy, a passionate AA advocate; how she had, however, slowly realized that the approach was not working (returners kept returning); and how she had recently been introduced to harm reduction.

She said she knew she should feel relief that she was being presented with an alternative to the hamster wheel she had been on with the patients. Instead, however, she just felt "drained" because, though she could conceptually understand harm reduction, she could not reconcile it with her deep-seated belief that substance use was wrong. "How," she asked, "does one do the mind shift from abstinence to harm reduction? How does one go from telling the patient that they need to stop using or they might die to telling the patient that if they are continuing their use they should do it responsibly so that they adhere to their treatment?" She described the first time she went into a session to present this new approach:

> So, I went into the session and I swallowed hard . . . I remember my exact words, "If you are going to use or you find yourself engaging in substance use, then do it responsibly so that you are still able to get to the clinic and take your treatment." I said it very fast to get it over and done with. . . . And I remember the response that I received. The patients just looked at me for a long while, shocked and confused at what I had said. They asked me how I could tell them that it was okay for them to use [substances] while they had TB and [were on] treatment. I then explained that their aim should focus on completing their treatment and not defaulting. So, if they were going to drink they should do it after going to the clinic and taking their tablets and drink responsibly to ensure that they are sober by the next morning to get to the clinic again.

She then spoke of how, even though she had subsequently noticed how her change in approach had resulted in a different, more positive dynamic developing between herself and patients in the hospital, she had struggled to write the presentation she was busy delivering. She had not known if she could stand up in front of people and lay claim to a perspective she still could not quite believe in. But then a few days before she had a moment of clarity: "We were preaching to them all the time that they needed to abstain, and if they didn't their TB would become resistant and they would die. I realized that we were actually telling them *what* to do, giving them the only solution [we could see] as health professionals, [and to be successful it required us to] change the world."

She spoke of realizing that her wish was impossible, out of line with the realities of the harsh lives patients lived. She spoke about how she realized that substance use played a role in people's lives:

> Their substances meant a lot to them. It made them feel better about themselves. It gave them a place in the world where they could fit in. And the reality of the situation is sad but true . . . we [health care providers] just cannot change the world. We cannot take away the hurt from the rape and abuse and the great need to belong somewhere. We [health care providers] just don't always have all the resources available. . . . [But] we can create an environment where [patients] are not being judged and labelled for being people that use substances, so that they can approach us and together we can find ways for them to cope through all their life struggles and difficulties to complete their treatment, be cured from TB, prevent drug-resistant TB and thus the spread of TB within our communities.

And then, ending on a soaring note of hope, she said, "Finally it makes some sense . . . we might just have the start of a new beginning."

Just over a year later, Soraya and I sat in her office in the hospital. Soraya had become head of occupational therapy for both the Cape Town TB hospitals. I had finished my research but was still returning to the hospital working with Soraya in the hope that we could get the rest of the hospital staff team to make the shift she had described in her presentation. With a colleague, I had just run a workshop in which we had tried to show how working from a place of moral judgment hindered treatment completion. We hit up against early resistance: a punitive approach to substance use (such as expulsion from the hospital) was described as more practical for hospital staff and nonusing patients. We had, however, started to see some changes in attitude, especially in senior staff, when we suggested that when there were problems, the focus should not be on substance use in and of itself, but rather on any behaviors, such as aggression or theft, that were encroaching on others. The nurses present were, however, clear that they were not moved. Soraya was disappointed. I was not, and I teasingly explained why: "Oh, I didn't expect a change in a day, it took six months of consistent work on you to get you to change!" Soraya chuckled and, in a show of generous self-criticism, acknowledged, "It did!" and then in a gentle joking indication that I was almost over the line of appropriate comment, she said, "You can go home now!" She was also, to some degree, indicating that I had done my job. She was not wrong. After that, I had little to do with the hospital, but five years later, as I was finishing writing this book, Soraya and I spoke over the phone. She had left DP Marais to become the deputy director of another hospital in the city, but the approach and program we set in place was still running in both hospitals. By that time, it was just accepted practice, even for the nurses.

ACKNOWLEDGMENTS

How does one account for the journey one has taken in developing a book? Mine, I think, started over twenty years ago, as I looked down on wheat-yellow hamlets on the banks of the Indus River in the Karakoram Highway, Pakistan, and realized that I wanted to better understand what shapes different ways of being in the world.

It was the Anthropology Department at the University of Cape Town—where I arrived a few months later and stayed for many years—that nurtured that desire. Fiona Ross, I couldn't have asked for a better teacher, guide, support, and friend through studies. I credit you with the development of my intellectual capacity a lot more than you know. (Sometimes when I relisten to my voice-files, I hear you in my own inflections and it makes me smile.) This book is only here because of your persistent insistence that it needed to exist. Susan Levine, your lectures pulled me into medical anthropology, and the time you took to gently persuade me to stay in the discipline when I was a wavering student served as an inflection point that kept me at the academy. Helen Macdonald, thank you for your insightful comments and suggestions and, as my co-supervisor, for always holding me to the standard you believed I could reach (even when I wasn't sure).

This ethnography owes most to those who generously shared and gave their time, space, and stories and managed my inquisitive presence. To the staff at the Delft South Matrix Clinic, thanks for your patience, assistance, guidance, and support. To the staff at DP Marais, I truly could not have done this without your warm, open welcome. Thank you for letting our relationship change from that of researcher and researched to colleagues and friends.

To my editor, Lenore Manderson, thank you for your rapid-fire faith in me, your inspiring mentorship, careful reading and editing, and your kindly critical eye over my work over the past six years. You tucked me under your wing when I needed it most and have been a phenomenal friend and support ever since I dropped you an email as an unknown student seeking some guidance. Margaret Ramsay, thank for your careful technical editing and indexing.

Nolwazi Mkhwanazi, how wonderful it is to say that anthropology stitched us together as friends sixteen years ago. I'm ever grateful for your continued encouragement and that you remain the person on the other end of the line (or glass of wine) when my ideas and thoughts need a solid, yet gentle sounding board.

Lindsey Reynolds, your extreme efficiency, intellectual generosity, and commitment to a practical social consciousness in all of your work remain completely inspiring. One day, perhaps I'll pull off some degree of emulation. Alison

Swartz, thanks for quiet, keyboard tapping times and lively conversations in PhD writing days.

To Daniel Jordan Smith, Jessaca Leinaweaver, Kay Warren, and all my fellow graduate students in the dissertators' writing group at Brown University, thank you so much for welcoming me into the Anthropology Department at Brown University; it was my semester there that kicked me back into a mode of reading critically and writing carefully.

To my friends and colleagues from TB HIV Care, your warmth, passion, and standards have been stretching and invigorating. I didn't even know the term "harm reduction" when you first heard about my work and offered support. Harry Hausler, thank you for your trust in my work before I knew its value. Shaun Shelly, your intellectual leadership and willingness to rock boats that needed capsizing have shaped my view of the world. Chapter 3 in this book owes everything to you. Andrew Scheibe, how I have valued the precision of your thought, even (perhaps especially) your ability to merge kindness with incisive critique. Andrew Lambert, you are the only person I know who could make me embarrassed about my lack of experience with brothels; thank you for including me in projects that pushed me into knowing what empathy for marginalized people really is. Katherine Young, your capacity for quietly providing the foundations of success for the people you work with is unparalleled.

Clémence Petit-Perrot and Guy Hubbard, you have been my rocks. I can only hope to be half as solid in my friendship in return. Keith Forces, thanks for teaching me to love and harness the wild wind, which proved a gift of joy and sanity. Lauren Biermann, your cheerleading and sage advice is always needed and appreciated. Debbie and Yair Schkolne, I doubt that this book would be here without the solidity of your friendship and supportive co-parenting.

This research would not have happened without the generous financial support I received from the David and Elaine Potter Foundation, the South African National Research Foundation, and the Max Lillie Sonnenberg Trust. My thanks to all who saw potential in me and to the University of Cape Town Postgraduate Funding Office. The staff there have provided excellent care and personalized support throughout my graduate studies.

And then, to the people of my heart and hearth: Libuseng Mutlanyane, thank you for keeping the children at bay so that I could sink into the deep focus needed for writing this book. My children, Ndalo and Anovuyo, thank you for allowing me all the chubby thigh squeezes that have kept me sane while writing this book during lockdown. To my husband, John Andrews, you arrived, with such certainty, at the perfect time. Finally, to my parents, my endless appreciation for teaching me to question, enquire, and figure things out for myself. It is a gift that keeps on giving.

NOTES

CHAPTER 1   RETURNERS

1. Treatment default was defined as treatment interruption "for two consecutive months or more during the treatment period" (Republic of South Africa 2014, 36). However, it was often more loosely used to indicate any periods of treatment interruption.

2. Tertiary hospitals are also called "acute" hospitals.

3. The reported cure rate for drug-sensitive TB increased to 78 percent in the 2016 Global Tuberculosis Report (World Health Organization 2016, 77).

4. Calculated using the WHO figure annual deaths in 2018 (World Health Organization 2018).

5. For example, disseminated TB, TB that is present in organs other than the lungs, almost exclusively develops in immune-suppressed patients.

6. See Chapters 3, 5, and 7.

7. The term "Coloured" has a specific South African meaning. During apartheid it was applied to anyone who was determined to be of a multiracial heritage. It has since become an identity, which some people ascribe to, others resist. However, it remains a category in the national census, and is in common usage.

8. This descriptive Afrikaans name translates to "Little tin town" in English.

9. This echoes critiques of apartheid-era forced removals in the 1980s (see Platsky and Walker 1985).

10. Tobacco barely enters my analysis, despite how common cigarette use is and its physiological impact. This is because tobacco use did not have a notable social impact on the ways in which TB treatment was given or received. While the doctors may have suggested to patients that they stop smoking, any concerted effort to persuade this was generally seen as a fight beyond the hospital staff's armory. Outside the women's ward, against the wall that caught the sun, single cigarettes would wend their ways through sociable patient groups on a sunny day.

11. At much the same time, a survey of the Stellenbosch district found that 9.5 percent of farms reported continued use of the dop system (Naude et al. 2003).

12. This has historically been a communally smoked pipe made from the neck of a broken bottle.

13. In 2014, 34 percent of people entering treatment centers reported tik as their primary drug of use (Dada et al. 2016, 5). Elsewhere in the country, alcohol is the most common substance reported at treatment centers.

14. See, for example, the work of Nicoli Nattrass (2007).

15. The Western Cape was, at the time, the only province not under the leadership of the African National Congress. This gave it some capacity to maneuver an alternative response to the national response.

16. Drug-resistant TB is any strain of the bacteria that has ceased to be susceptible to (killed by) one or more of the drugs used for treatment. There is no uniformity to drug resistance—strains of TB can be resistant to more than one of the medications usually used.

17. Capreomycin, kanamycin, and amikacin.

18. This varied somewhat according to weight.

19. Bharat Venkat (2016) has illustrated how the concept of cure as a stable condition resulting from effective treatment is itself constructed, unstable, and challenged by infection relapse.

20. The institution was initially known as Princess Alice Home of Recovery and housed only forty beds (Louw 1979).
21. Sunlight kills TB bacilli and wind disperses it, reducing the concentration in the air.
22. Seventy percent of these HIV-positive patients were not taking ARVs when they arrived at the hospital. Almost 60 percent of these had started on ARVs at least once. Those who had never taken ARVs were divided between those who were not yet deemed sick enough for this treatment to have started (the minority) and those who had only recently found out their HIV-positive status.
23. This recognition that people did not always want to engage with me meant that I was particularly careful to assess willingness to talk in body language and approach, as much as I did in the processes of informed consent, which I undertook as a standard part of this research.
24. See Chapter 6.
25. See Chapter 2.
26. Aaron Goodfellow (2008) points out, in relation to methamphetamine, that the line between substances regarded as therapeutic and substances regarded as dangerous becomes even fuzzier if we take a historical perspective.
27. See Chapter 2.
28. I did not, in fact, collect information on racial demographic during my research; though in both facilities, information on race was collected, this was on the assessment of the staff based on name, language, and skin tone, rather than the self-description of the attendee. My comments here are, then, based on my own, similarly problematic assessments.

CHAPTER 2   THE STICKINESS OF MORAL OPINION

1. The Step Up Project is coordinated by TB/HIV Care Association. See www.tbhivcare.org.
2. The population Officer P was talking about was very largely White, so this was not veiled racism.
3. See, for example, http://www.surgeon-and-safari.co.za/. Similarly, "Stepping Stones Rehab Center" is listed as a "luxury rehab," and the homepage says, "This well-established center located in a seaside village of Cape Town has a reputation for top-notch treatment, attracting clients from around the world."
4. https://www.akeso.co.za/clinic/Akeso-Stepping-Stones
5. This totaled 6,954 in the Western Cape in 2014, inclusive of retreatment (Dada et al. 2016).
6. http://www.aasouthafrica.org.za/Meetings.aspx
7. I discuss appeals to evidence later in this chapter.
8. See American Psychiatric Association (2013).
9. This was the framing presented in the Delft Matrix Clinic.
10. Also referred to as "addiction subjectivities" by Summerson Carr (2013).
11. See also Bourgois (1995).
12. Something I turn to in Chapter 4.
13. See https://www.brucekalexander.com/articles-speeches/rat-park/282-rat-park-versus-the-new-york-times-2
14. This is supposed to happen every five years. In reality, release dates have been rather more flexible.
15. This has uncomfortable echoes of the early response to the AIDS epidemic, where in South Africa, abstinence was the first pillar of prevention, which, because of its impossibility, resulted in the death of millions.
16. These include "gender, sex, marital status, ethnic or social origin, colour, sexual orientation, age, disability, religion, conscience, belief, culture, language or birth, amongst others."

17. A poll of youth in 2013 indicated that three-quarters of the participants wanted the death penalty reinstated. https://www.timeslive.co.za/news/south-africa/2013-02-22-bring -back-death-penalty-survey/

18. The *Diagnostic and Statistical Manual of Mental Disorders* periodically put out by the American Psychiatric Association.

19. The insertion of moral judgments in efforts to control and contain TB has a long history. Robert Koch's 1882 discovery of the tubercle bacillus ushered in a new era of public health in America, in which "clean living" (a euphemism in part for the avoidance from alcohol) was emphasized (Rothman 1995, 183). Alcohol use was seen as a "personal vice" that distinguished those who used it from the innocent poor, who were suffering the consequences of circumstance (1995, 184). Around the same time, in France, alcoholism, syphilis, and the perceived moral depravity of the working classes were causally linked to TB disease (Barnes 1995).

CHAPTER 3   CO-CONSTITUTIONS

1. I do not describe any of the doctors in any detail in order to avoid easy identification, though they will likely be identifiable to those who know the hospital well.

2. This conversation occurred entirely in Afrikaans. I have translated here for ease of reading.

3. See Chapter 5 for more on Wendy's role in the hospital.

4. Homelands were portions of land designated "independent" (but only recognized as such by the South African government) as part of the South African project of racial segregation.

5. Up until twelve weeks, pregnancy termination has been available free of charge in the public health care sector since 1996, but as a government service, it is not always easy to access, and waiting times may make it an impossible option.

6. It was unclear to me (and perhaps to her) when she had acquired HIV.

7. Babalwa did not report whether her child was born with any obvious signs of fetal alcohol syndrome.

8. The 2013–2014 child support grant was R290 (approximately $29) for April to September 2013 and R300 (approximately $30) for October 2013 to March 2014, respectively (Berry et al. 2013, 92).

9. This is a diagnostic test "that can be used with minimal technical expertise, enabling rapid diagnosis of TB and simultaneous assessment of rifampicin resistance within 2 hours" (Zumla, Nahid, and Cole 2013, 389). However, the test does not distinguish between live and dead bacilli (Republic of South Africa 2014).

10. Newer diagnostic procedures, such as urine tests, are now also being developed, but these have yet to hit widescale rollout in any country.

11. Artificial intelligence is increasingly being used to increase diagnostic accuracy, but in 2014, this was brand-new technology still being presented at conferences to the consternation of some health care providers.

12. In contrast, I know of an elderly middle-class man whose TB escaped detection despite standard symptoms for many months because TB was not even considered in the diagnostic options because it is seen to be a disease of the poor.

13. For a historical description of how the individual body became the place of enquiry for understanding disease, see Michel Foucault's defining book, *The Birth of the Clinic* (1973).

14. Felicity reappears in Chapter 7, where I discuss the multiple kinds of care the hospital seeks to provide.

15. Despite its top-rated status as an infectious disease killer, TB has failed to garner much attention (and funding), relative to other communicable diseases.

16. The BCG vaccine is provided to all infants in South Africa.

17. For a beautiful description of the ways in which doctors in a hospital in Papua New Guinea similarly make decisions through doubt, and tinker in the hope of hitting on effective treatment, see Alice Street (2014).

18. As with randomized controlled trials, context is being removed, when context is what matters (Adams 2013).

19. The most notable clarifications of the term are provided in Singer (2009) and Singer and Clair (2003).

20. "AIDS"—acquired immune deficiency syndrome—was named before the virus that caused the illness was discovered. Consequently, unlike TB, where the pathogen and the illness have the same name, two separate names were used. However, given the nebulousness of the differences between a state of infection and illness, this differentiation has dropped from common use in medical literature.

21. More recently, Singer and colleagues define syndemics as "the aggregation of two or more diseases or other health conditions in a population in which there is some level of deleterious biological or behavior interface that exacerbates the negative health effects of any or all of the diseases involved" (Singer et al. 2017). The complexity of this newer definition does not, unfortunately, make it any more practical for my purposes.

22. This does not mean that people around the sick do not suspect TB. I was told numerous times by people that they thought their friends, with whom they had regular use patterns, had TB.

23. Though recently acknowledged (Singer, Bulled, and Ostrach 2020), this is currently not a focus of syndemics literature.

24. This is the approach of much traditional health care practice in South Africa and the reason why many people continue to seek out the services of traditional providers, even if they have a belief in the science of biomedicine.

CHAPTER 4   SALIENCE AND SILENCE

1. Bureaucratic writing, such as the recordkeeping required by frontline health care workers, has long been seen as instruments of power, a way of states exerting control over citizens (Hull 2012).

2. This has echoes of recorded responses of police not filing cases they know will be hard to follow up as this can affect their conviction rates (Commission of Inquiry into Allegations of Police Inefficiency and a Breakdown in Relations Between SAPS and the Community in Khayelitsha 2014, see http://www.khayelitshacommission.org.za/final-report.html).

3. This was a figure inclusive of alcohol, but exclusive of cigarettes, which were not really discussed as a substance of abuse, though their damage to the lungs was recognized. See Chapter 2.

4. All these folders without information were from patients in Ward 5, where the doctor relied on the occupational therapy team and the social workers to do these assessments. It is likely that these patients were either too sick for these to be done or were only in the hospital for a short period and left before the team were able to do them.

5. These figures also need to be interpreted in light of the fact that mandrax is always smoked in combination with dagga. The 10.8 percent of patients who smoked mandrax would all also have smoked dagga.

6. The reason for this discrepancy between treatment center data and hospital data is unclear, although in my earlier work, I showed that women were particularly reluctant to report to treatment centers compared to men (Versfeld 2012). This may result in underreporting at treatment centers.

7. See Lucinda in Chapter 3.

8. Social workers would sometimes also gather detailed information about substance use in conversations that were structured as counseling sessions, but (following the logic of counseling and privacy) notes about these were devoid of detail. "Substance abuse tik" might be the extent of the inscription after a long discussion about a chaotic home environment and family-wide substance use.

9. I do not know whether there were temporal limitations to this, for example, whether drinking was only done in the evenings.

10. See Chapter 3.

11. Three-quarters of these early leavers were still smear positive (that is, likely to be infectious) in their last tests, and 94 percent of the smear-positive leavers were people who used substances.

CHAPTER 5   THE CHALLENGE OF "UNRULY" PATIENTS

1. Mila did far more than this. She kept track of patients, greeting them by name and commenting on what was next due for their treatment process—a sputum sample, perhaps, or a drug regime change—when they came into the clinic. Patients trusted her to ensure their care followed the correct path, and they often sought her out first. Mila also oversaw the DOTS supporters who kept a daily eye on patients taking treatment "in community," and she acted as a DOTS supporter for four patients herself. It was a job of pitiful financial reward—R600 (approximately $43) per month. "I don't think anyone would do this for the money," she wryly observed, though later conversations indicated just how important this small income was to her family.

2. This reluctance to treat the unruly patient needs to be understood not only in terms of the tyranny of numbers but also in the larger national and international context of concern about the growing epidemic of drug-resistant TB; this is something I turn to later in this chapter.

3. Harper (2005, 2006) shows that this is exactly what happened in Nepal. The categorization required in the implementation of DOTS resulted in the exclusion of those patients who did not fit neatly into categories and therefore fell outside of frameworks for reporting.

4. Children—due to their still establishing immune systems—are particularly susceptible to becoming ill with TB if they are exposed. National Tuberculosis Management Guidelines (2014) therefore require that children who have had close exposure to active TB should take a six-month course of prophylaxis.

5. On seeing them, I immediately had a nagging worry about the exposure to TB that the children, so young and therefore very vulnerable to infection, were receiving. On hearing this narrative, I realized that my concerns were rendered irrelevant in the face of the action they were taking due to their worries about exposure in the home.

6. Given that MDR TB does not convert to drug-sensitive TB on treatment, this implies reinfection.

7. I was not able to ascertain why Aafiyah was powerless to stop her ex-husband entering the house without recourse to other authorities. My suspicion was that he was the leaseholder to the house. In exceedingly resource-constrained settings where housing was in short supply, this would explain Aafiyah's limited power.

8. For a similar description of narrative crafting in appeal for state support (though the crafting is done by a third party), see Giordano (2015).

9. See www.tbhivcare.org

10. The tool allowed for more careful collection of substance use data in patients than the folders allowed.

11. At the time of my folder review, 72 percent of patients in the hospital were referred from hospitals, whereas 28 percent of patients had been referred from clinics. This was, by the doctors' reckoning, a fairly standard breakdown.

CHAPTER 6   CARE TO CURE

1. For an examination of tinkering in TB care provision, see Helen Macdonald's description of care provision in India (Macdonald 2020).
2. For a discussion about the extent to which responsibilization actually manifests in South African HIV care, see Christopher Colvin and colleagues (Colvin, Robins, and Leavens 2010).
3. For a South African example of this playing out at the level of treatment provision, see Vale and colleagues' description of regimes of ART provision and control in youth (Vale et al. 2017).
4. Sometimes patients arrived back at the hospital on Tuesday or Wednesday. When this happened, they were sent back home.
5. South Africa has an extensive system of social welfare grants. These include "disability grants," which are given to anyone who is unable to work due to mental or physical disability that impairs that person's capacity to work for six months or longer (see the government website: http://www.gov.za/services/social-benefits/disability-grant). I discuss the hospital's support in attaining social grants for certain patients in more detail in Chapter 8.
6. "Shebeen" is a South African term for a place where alcohol is sold and consumed. There was an informal shebeen on the other side of the fence at one of the corners of the hospital grounds.
7. See Chapter 8 discussions about patients' fear of leaving and the conclusion for a critique of the ways in which the hospital generated this fear.
8. Sputum conversion means that the sputum no longer had infectious bacilli.
9. FAS is a consequence of high levels of alcohol exposure in utero. It leads to specific facial features and can include learning difficulties and poor motor control, among other things. Some areas in the Western Cape have the highest recorded levels of FAS in the world (Viljoen et al. 2005; May et al. 2000).
10. Thirty-nine percent of patients in the hospital at the time of my folder review were recorded to be experiencing at least their second episode of TB. One female patient in DP Marais was being treated for the twelfth time when I met her. After her discharge, we met again at the Delft South clinic. She explained to me that she lived with an uncle who had been ill with TB for years and refused treatment. She died shortly afterward.
11. This potential was not always realized. Sometimes answers did not appear. Moreover, these bedside visits were also sometimes the time in which a decision would be made that ongoing care would be palliative, though hints of this were only to be found in the ways in which communication closed into the whispers of the clustered group of doctors.
12. TB meningitis occurs when the bacilli seed into the brain meninges.
13. The danger of death is a commonly used persuasive device when it comes to TB treatment. It assumes, of course, that the patient wants to live, which was certainly not always the case.
14. Second-line ARV treatment is the medicine regime given when the most commonly taken standardized medications are no longer suppressing HIV. As with second-line TB treatment, it includes a different range of medications.
15. Occasional weekend home visits were allowed once the patient was seen to be stable. This was usually after the first two months in the hospital.

16. Marlow's mother, similarly unhappy, visited the hospital some weeks later to challenge their decision to discharge him.

CHAPTER 7   CATCHING BREATH

1. Similarly, writing about health care provision waiting rooms, Catherine Burns has described these spaces as a "liminal place, a place in-between, a place of ritualized passivity, dependent on the co-operation of patient, the supplicant"(Burns 2014).
2. Abney (2014) describes a similar parsing of life circulating in Brooklyn Chest Hospital.
3. *Papa* and *Oupa* are Afrikaans terms both used widely for grandfather.
4. See Chapter 6.
5. It could have been that Tammy's friend had both drug-sensitive and drug-resistant TB, and she only contracted the drug-sensitive strain.
6. This contrasted to the disclosure creep I wrote about in Chapter 5. Joseph and Tammy show that sometimes disclosure was less about the generation of trust and more about a rupture of confidence brought on by an impending discharge from the hospital.
7. Kelly Ray Knight (2015) provides another example of the requirement of abstinence thwarting stated goals. She writes about how addicted pregnant women were required to be abstinent in order to access housing, which resulted in additional rather than reduced precarity and risk to the fetus.
8. Heroin use can result in constricted pupils that do not respond to changes in light.
9. The minimum monthly wage at the time for domestic work was R1877.70/$188 (see www.labour.gov.za).

CHAPTER 8   ANTHROPOLOGY IN ACTION

1. I knew about Jeffrey's changed life circumstances because, with his permission, I had stayed in contact with his mother.
2. Information available, however, does indicate that there are concerns about combining HIV and hepatitis C medication with methamphetamine (Bruce, Altice, and Friedland 2008).
3. The fact that I had worked around substance use for years prior in South Africa without having come across the term "harm reduction" indicates the degree to which this was a minority perspective.

REFERENCES

Abney, Kate. 2014. "At the Foot of Table Mountain: Paediatric Tuberculosis Patient Experiences in a Centralised Treatment Facility in Cape Town, South Africa." Unpublished doctoral thesis. University of Cape Town.

Adams, Vincanne. 2013. "Evidence-Based Global Public Health." In *When People Come First: Critical Studies in Global Health*, edited by João Guilherme Biehl and Adriana Petryna, 54–90. Princeton, NJ: Princeton University Press.

Adichie, Chimamanda Ngozi. 2009. "The Danger of a Single Story." *Ted Talks*. TED Global Talks.

Alexander, Bruce. 2010. *The Globalization of Addiction: A Study in Poverty of the Spirit*. Oxford: Oxford University Press.

Alexander, Bruce K., Barry L. Beyerstein, Patricia F. Hadaway, and Robert B. Coambs. 1981. "Effect of Early and Later Colony Housing on Oral Ingestion of Morphine in Rats." *Pharmacology, Biochemistry and Behavior* 15 (4): 571–576. https://doi.org/10.1016/0091 -3057(81)90211-2.

American Psychiatric Association. 2013. "Substance-Related and Addictive Disorders." In *Diagnostic and Statistical Manual of Mental Disorders: DSM-5*, 481–589. Washington, D.C.: American Psychiatric Association. https://doi.org/10.1176/appi.books.9780890425596.190656.

Atkins, Salla, David Biles, Simon Lewin, Karin Ringsberg, and Anna Thorson. 2010. "Patients' Experiences of an Intervention to Support Tuberculosis Treatment Adherence in South Africa." *Journal of Health Services Research & Policy* 15 (3): 163–170. https://doi.org/10.1258 /jhsrp.2010.009111.

Atkins, Salla, Simon Lewin, Karin C. Ringsberg, and Anna Thorson. 2012. "Towards an Empowerment Approach in Tuberculosis Treatment in Cape Town, South Africa: A Qualitative Analysis of Programmatic Change." *Global Health Action* 5: 1–12.

Barnes, David S. 1995. *The Making of a Social Disease*. Berkeley: University of California Press.

Bateman, Chris. 2006a. "Living the TB Resistance Nighmare." *South African Medical Journal* 96 (10): 55–56.

———. 2006b. "'Tik' Causing a Public Health Crisis." *South African Medical Journal* 96 (8): 28–29.

———. 2007. "'One Shot' to Kill MDR TB—Or Risk Patient Death." *South African Medical Journal* 97 (12): 1233–1236.

———. 2015. "Tugela Ferry's Extensively Drug-Resistant Tuberculosis—10 Years On." *South African Medical Journal* 105 (7): 517–520. https://doi.org/10.7196/SAMJnew.7838.

Béhague, Dominique Pareja, Helen Gonçalves, and Cesar Gomes Victora. 2009. "Anthropology and Epidemiology: Learning Epistemological Lessons through a Collaborative Venture." *Ciencia & Saude Coletiva* 13 (6): 1701–1710. https://doi.org/10.1590/S1413 -81232008000600002.

Benton, Adia. 2012. "Exceptional Suffering? Enumeration and Vernacular Accounting in the HIV-Positive Experience." *Medical Anthropology* 31 (4): 310–328. https://doi.org/10.1080 /01459740.2011.631959.

Berry, Lizette, Linda Biersteker, Andrew Dawes, Lori Lake, and Charmaine Smith. 2013. *The South African Child Gauge*. Cape Town: Children's Institute, University of Cape Town.

http://www.ci.uct.ac.za/sites/default/files/image_tool/images/367/Child_Gauge
/South_African_Child_Gauge_2013/SouthAfricanChildGauge2013.pdf.

Bhardwaj, Anvita, and Brandon A. Kohrt. 2020. "Syndemics of HIV with Mental Illness and Other Noncommunicable Diseases: A Research Agenda to Address the Gap between Syndemic Theory and Current Research Practice." *PMC* 15 (4): 226–231. https://doi.org/10.1097/COH.0000000000000627.

Biehl, João. 2005. "Technologies of Invisibility." In *Anthropologies of Modernity Foucault, Governmentality, and Life Politics*, edited by Jonathan Xavier Inda, Oxford, 248–271. Oxford: Blackwell Press.

Biehl, João Guilherme. 2005. *Vita: Life in a Zone of Social Abandonment*. Berkeley: University of California Press.

Biruk, Crystal. 2018. *Cooking Data: Culture and Politics in an African Research World*. Durham, NC: Duke University Press.

Bourgois, Philippe. 1995. *In Search of Respect: Selling Crack in El Barrio*. Cambridge: Cambridge University Press.

———. 2002. "Anthropology and Epidemiology on Drugs: The Challenges of Cross-Methodological and Theoretical Dialogue." *International Journal of Drug Policy* 13 (4): 259–269. https://doi.org/10.1016/S0955-3959(02)00115-9.

Bourgois, Philippe, Mark Lettiere, James Quesada, and San Francisco. 1997. "Social Misery and the Sanctions of Substance Abuse: Confronting HIV Risk among Homeless Heroin Addicts in San Francisco." *Social Problems* 44 (2): 155–173.

Bourgois, Philippe, and Jeff Schonberg. 2009. *Righteous Dopefiend*. Berkeley: University of California Press.

Briggs, Charles L., and Clara Mantini-Briggs. 2003. *Stories in the Time of Cholera: Racial Profiling during a Medical Nightmare*. Berkeley: University of California Press.

Brives, Charlotte, Frédéric Le Marcis, and Emilia Sanabria. 2016. "What's in a Context? Tenses and Tensions in Evidence-Based Medicine." *Medical Anthropology: Cross-Cultural Studies in Health and Illness* 35 (5): 369–376. https://doi.org/10.1080/01459740.2016.1160089.

Brown, Ryan. 2010. "Crystal Methamphetamine Use among American Indian and White Youth in Appalachia: Social Context, Masculinity, and Desistance." *Addiction Research and Theory* 18 (3): 250–269.

Bruce, R. D., F. L. Altice, and G. H. Friedland. 2008. "Pharmacokinetic Drug Interactions Between Drugs of Abuse and Antiretroviral Medications: Implications and Management for Clinical Practice." *Expert Review of Clinical Pharmacology* 1 (1): 115–127. https://doi.org/10.1586/17512433.1.1.115.

Bruce, R. Douglas, Barrot Lambdin, Olivia Chang, Frank Masao, Jessie Mbwambo, Ibrahim Mteza, Cassian Nyandindi, et al. 2014. "Lessons from Tanzania on the Integration of HIV and Tuberculosis Treatments into Methadone Assisted Treatment." *International Journal on Drug Policy* 25 (1): 22–25. https://doi.org/10.1016/j.drugpo.2013.09.005.

Buchanan, Julian. 2004. "Tackling Problem Drug Use." *Social Work in Mental Health* 2 (2–3): 117–138. https://doi.org/10.1300/J200v02n02.

Burns, Catherine. 2014. "Patience in the Waiting Room—the Doctor Will See You Just Now." *Mail and Guardian*, 6 October.

Campbell, Nancy D. 2013. "'Why Can't They Stop?' A Highly Public Misunderstanding of Science." In *Addiction Trajectories*, edited by Eugene Raikhel and William Garriott, 238–262. Durham, NC: Duke University Press.

Campbell, Nancy D., and Susan J. Shaw. 2008. "Incitements to Discourse: Illicit Drugs, Harm Reduction, and the Production of Ethnographic Subjects." *Cultural Anthropology* 23 (4): 688–717. https://doi.org/10.1111/j.1548-1360.2008.00023.x.

Carr, Summerson. 2010. *Scripting Addiction: The Politics of Therapeutic Talk and American Sobriety*. Princeton, NJ: Princeton University Press.

———. 2013. "Signs of Sobriety: Rescripting American Addiction Counselling." In *Addiction Trajectories*, edited by Eugene Raikhel and William Garriott, 160–187. Durham, NC: Duke University Press.

Carroll, Jennifer. 2011. "A Woman among Addicts: The Production and Management of Identities in a Ukrainian Harm Reduction Program." *Anthropology of Eastern Europe* 29 (1): 23–34.

———. 2013. *Barriers to Treatment Adherence in Ukrainian Tuberculosis Control Programs*. Research brief. IREX. https://www. irex. org/sites/default/files/Carroll% 20Research% 20Brief.

Chapple, A., S. Ziebland, and A. McPherson. 2004. "Stigma, Shame, and Blame Experienced by Patients with Lung Cancer: Qualitative Study." *British Medical Journal* 328 (7454): 1470–1473. https://doi.org/10.1136/bmj.38111.639734.7c.

Churchyard, G. J., L. D. Mametja, L. Mvusi, N. Ndjeka, A. C. Hessling, A. Reid, S. Babatunde, and Y. Pillay. 2014. "Tuberculosis Control in South Africa: Successes, Challenges and Recommendations." *South African Medical Journal* 104 (3): 1–3. https://doi.org/10.7196/SAMJ.7689.

Cock, Jacqueline. 1989. *Maid and Madams: Domestic Workers Under Apartheid*. London: The Women's Press.

Colvin, Christopher, Steven Robins, and Joan Leavens. 2010. "Grounding 'Responsibilisation Talk': Masculinities, Citizenship and HIV in Cape Town, South Africa." *Journal of Development Studies* 46 (7): 1179–1195. https://doi.org/10.1080/00220388.2010.487093.

Cramm, Jane M., Harry J. M. Finkenflügel, Valerie Møller, and Anna P. Nieboer. 2010. "TB Treatment Initiation and Adherence in a South African Community Influenced More by Perceptions than by Knowledge of Tuberculosis." *BCM Public Health* 10 (72). pmid:20163702. https://doi.org/10.1186/1471-2458-10-72.

Dada, Siphokazi, Nadine Burnhams Harker, Yolanda Williams, Jodilee Erasmus, Charles Parry, Arvin Bhana, Erika Nel, Diana Kitshoff, Roger Weimann, and David Fourie. 2015. *Monitoring Alcohol and Drug Use Treatment Admissions in South Africa*: Phase 37. SACENDU. https://www.samrc.ac.za/sites/default/files/attachments/2016-06-28/SacenduReport June2015.pdf.

Dada, Siphokazi, Jodilee Erasmus, Nadine Harker Burnhams, Charles Parry, Arvin Bhana, Furzana Timol, and David Fourie. 2016. *Monitoring Alcohol and Drug Use Treatment Admissions in South Africa*: Phase 39. SACENDU. https://www.samrc.ac.za/sites/default/files /attachments/2016-10-17/SACENDUPhase39.pdf.

Dada, Siphokazi, Nadine Harker, Burnhams Jodilee, Erasmus Warren, Charles Parry, Arvin Bhana, Sandra Pretorius, et al. 2019. *Monitoring Alcohol and Drug Use Treatment Admissions in South Africa*: Phase 44. SACENDU. https://www.samrc.ac.za/sites/default/files /attachments/2019-04-30/SACENDUFullReportPhase44.pdf.

de Certeau, Michel. 1984. *The Practice of Everyday Life. The Practice of Everyday Life*. Berkeley, CA: University of California Press.

Deiss, Robert G., Timothy C. Rodwell, and Richard S. Garfein. 2009. "Tuberculosis and Illicit Drug Use: Review and Update." *Clinical Infectious Diseases* 48 (1): 72–82. https://doi.org /10.1086/594126.

Department of Social Development, Central Drug Authority. 2013. *National Drug Master Plan 2013–2017*. Pretoria: Department of Social Development.

Department of Welfare, Drug Advisory Board. 1999. *National Drug Master Plan*. Pretoria: Department of Welfare.

Engelmann, Lukas, and Janina Kehr. 2015. "Double Trouble? Towards an Epistemology of Co-Infection." *Medicine Anthropology Theory* 2 (1): 1–31.

Erikson, Susan L. 2012. "Global Health Business: The Production and Performativity of Statistics in Sierra Leone and Germany." *Medical Anthropology* 31 (4): 367–384. https://doi.org /10.1080/01459740.2011.621908.

Farmer, Paul. 1992. *AIDS and Accusation: Haiti and the Geography of Blame.* Berkeley: University of California Press.

———. 1997. "Social Scientists and the New Tuberculosis." *Social Science & Medicine* 44 (3): 347–358.

Farmer, Paul, and Edward Nardell. 1998. "Editorial: Nihilism and Pragmatism in Tuberculosis Control." *American Journal of Public Health* 7 (July): 1014–1016.

Fassin, Didier. 2007. *When Bodies Remember: Experiences and Politics of AIDS in South Africa.* San Francisco: University of California Press.

Foucault, Michel. 1973. *The Birth of the Clinic: An Archaeology of Medical Perception.* London: Travistock.

———. 2003. *The Essential Foucault: Selections from Works of Foucault, 1954–1984.* Edited by Paul Rose and Nikolas Rabinow. New York: New Press.

Friedman, L. N., G. S. Sullivan, R. P. Bevilaqua, and R. Loscos. 1987. "Tuberculosis Screening in Alcoholics and Drug Addicts." *American Review of Respiratory Disease* 136 (5): 1188–1193.

Gaede, B. M. 2016. "Doctors as Street-Level Bureaucrats in a Rural Hospital in South Africa." *Rural and Remote Health* 16 (3461): 1–9.

Garcia, Angela. 2008. "The Elegiac Addict: History, Chronicity, and the Melancholic Subject." *Cultural Anthropology* 23 (4): 718–746. https://doi.org/10.1111/j.1548-1360.2008.00024.x.

———. 2010. *The Pastoral Clinic: Addiction and Dispossession along the Rio Grande.* Berkeley: University of California Press. https://doi.org/10.1007/s13398-014-0173-7.2.

Garriott, William. 2013. "'You Can Always Tell Who's Using Meth': Methamphetamine Addiction and the Semiotics of Criminal Difference." In *Addiction Trajectories*, edited by Eugene Raikhel and William Garriott. Durham, NC: Duke University Press. 213–237.

Getahun, Haileyesus, Annabel Baddeley, and Mario Raviglione. 2013. "Managing Tuberculosis in People Who Use and Inject Illicit Drugs." *Bulletin of the World Health Organization* 91 (2): 154–156. https://doi.org/10.2471/BLT.13.117267.

Gibson, Diana. 2004. "The Gaps in the Gaze in South African Hospitals." *Social Science and Medicine* 59 (10): 2013–2024. https://doi.org/10.1016/j.socscimed.2004.03.006.

Giordano, Cristiana. 2015. "Lying the Truth." *Current Anthropology* 56 (December): S211–S221. https://doi.org/10.1086/683272.

Goodfellow, Aaron. 2008. "Pharmaceutical Intimacy: Sex, Death, and Methamphetamine." *Home Cultures* 5 (3): 271–300.

Gould, Chandré, and Peter Folb. 2002. *Project Coast: Apartheid's Chemical and Biological Warfare Programme.* NIDIR. https://unidir.org/publication/project-coast-apartheids -chemical-and-biological-warfare-programme.

Grelotti, David J., Elizabeth F. Closson, Jennifer A. Smit, Zonke Mabude, Lynn T. Matthews, Steven A. Safren, David R. Bangsberg, and Matthew J. Mimiaga. 2014. "Whoonga: Potential Recreational Use of HIV Antiretroviral Medication in South Africa." *AIDS and Behavior* 18 (3): 511–518. https://doi.org/10.1007/s10461-013-0575-0.

Gundersen, Storla Dag, Solomon Yimer, and Gunnar Aksel Bjune. 2008. "A Systematic Review of Delay in the Diagnosis and Treatment of Tuberculosis." *BMC Public Health* 8 (15). https://doi.org/10.1186/1471-2458-8-15.

Gupta, A., J. Mbwambo, I. Mteza, S. Shenoi, B. Lambdin, C. Nyandindi, B. I. Doula, S. Mfaume, and R. Douglas Bruce. 2014. "Active Case Finding for Tuberculosis among People Who Inject Drugs on Methadone Treatment in Dar Es Salaam, Tanzania." *International Journal of Tuberculosis and Lung Disease* 18 (7): 793–798. https://doi.org/10.5588/ijtld.13.0208.

Hacking, Ian. 1990. *The Taming of Chance*. Cambridge: Cambridge University Press.

Hall, Wayne, Adrian Carter, and Cynthia Forlini. 2015. "The Brain Disease Model of Addiction: Is It Supported by the Evidence and Has It Delivered on Its Promises?" *The Lancet Psychiatry* 2 (1): 105–110. https://doi.org/10.1016/S2215-0366(14)00126-6.

Hammer, Rachel, Molly Dingel, Jenny Ostergren, Brad Partridge, Jennifer McCormick, and Barbara A. Koenig. 2013. "Addiction: Current Criticism of the Brain Disease Paradigm." *AJOB Neuroscience* 4 (3): 27–32. https://doi.org/10.1080/21507740.2013.796328.

Han, Clara. 2011. "Symptoms of Another Life: Time, Possibility, and Domestic Relations in Chile's Credit Economy." *Cultural Anthropology* 26 (1): 7–32. https://doi.org/10.1111/j.1548-1360.2010.01078.x.

Hansen, Helena. 2013. "Pharmaceutical Evangelism and Spiritual Capital: An American Tale of Two Communities of Addicted Selves." In *Addiction Trajectories*, edited by Eugene Raikhel and William Garriott, 108–125. Durham, NC: Duke University Press.

Harper, Ian. 2005. "Interconnected and Inter-Infected: DOTS and the Stabilisation of the Tuberculosis Control Programme in Nepal." In *The Aid Effect: Giving and Governing in International Development*, edited by David Mosse and David Lewis, 126–149. London: Pluto Press.

———. 2006. "Anthropology, DOTS and Understanding Tuberculosis Control in Nepal." *Journal of Biosocial Science* 38 (1): 57–67. https://doi.org/10.1017/S0021932005000982.

———. 2010. "Extreme Condition, Extreme Measures? Compliance, Drug Resistance, and the Control of Tuberculosis." *Anthropology & Medicine* 17 (2): 201–214. https://doi.org/10.1080/13648470.2010.493606.

Haysom, Simone. 2019. *Hiding in Plain Sight: Heroin's Stealthy Takeover of South Africa*. Policy Brief. ENACT. https://enactafrica.org/research/policy-briefs/hiding-in-plain-sight-heroins-stealthy-takeover-of-south-africa.

Haysom, Simone, Peter Gastrow, and Mark Shaw. 2018. *The Heroin Coast: A Political Economy along the Eastern Africa Seaboard*. Research Paper. ENACT. https://globalinitiative.net/wp-content/uploads/2018/07/2018-06-27-research-paper-heroin-coast-pdf.pdf.

Heim, Derek. 2014. "Addiction: Not Just a Brain Malfunction." *Nature* 507 (7490): 40. https://doi.org/10.1038/507040a.

Heller, T., R. J. Lessells, C. G. Wallrauch, T. Bärnighausen, G. S. Cooke, L. Mhlongo, I. Master, and M. L. Newell. 2010. "Community-Based Treatment for Multidrug-Resistant Tuberculosis in Rural KwaZulu-Natal, South Africa." *International Journal of Tuberculosis and Lung Disease* 14 (4): 420–426.

Henderson, Patricia C. 2011. *A Kinship of Bones: AIDS, Intimacy and Care in Rural KwaZulu-Natal*. Amsterdam: Amsterdam University Press.

Heywood, Mark. 2009. "South Africa's Treatment Action Campaign: Combining Law and Social Mobilization to Realize the Right to Health." *Journal of Human Rights Practice* 1 (1): 14–36. https://doi.org/10.1093/jhuman/hun006.

Holtz, T. H., J. Lancaster, K. F. Laserson, C. D. Wells, L. Thorpe, K. Weyer, and Tuberculosis Elimination, and Disease Control. 2006. "Risk Factors Associated with Default from Multidrug-Resistant Tuberculosis Treatment, South Africa, 1999–2001." *International Journal of Tuberculosis and Lung Disease* 10 (6): 649–655.

Howell, Simon, and Katherine Couzyn. 2015. "The South African National Drug Master Plan 2013–2017: A Critical Review." *South African Journal of Criminal Justice* 28 (August): 1–23.

Hull, Matthew S. 2012. *Government of Paper*. Berkeley: University of California Press.

Human, Oliver. 2011. "The Rings around Jonathan's Eyes: HIV/AIDS Medicine at the Margins of Administration." *Medical Anthropology* 30 (2): 222–239. https://doi.org/10.1080/01459740.2011.552452.

Human Sciences Research Council of South Africa. 2010. *Tsireledzani: Understanding the Dimensions of Human Trafficking in Southern Africa*. National Prosecuting Authority of South Africa. https://www.activateleadership.co.za/wp-content/uploads/2020/03/understanding-dimentions-of-Human-trafficking-in-South-Africa.pdf.

Inciardi, James A., and Lana D. Harrison. 1999. "Introduction: The Concept of Harm Reduction." In *Harm Reduction: National and International Perspectives*, edited by James A. Inciardi and Lana D. Harrison. Thousand Oaks, CA: Sage.

Jain, Lochlann. 2013. *Malignant: How Cancer Becomes Us*. Berkeley: University of California Press.

Jain, Lochlann, and Sharon Kaufman. 2011. "Introduction to Special Issue after Progress: Time and Improbable Futures in Clinic Spaces." *Medical Anthropology Quarterly* 25 (2): 183–188.

Jooste, Bronwyn. 2011. "Drug Abuse at 'Crisis Levels' in the Cape." *Cape Argus*, 12 August.

KCOI (Khayelitsha Commission of Inquiry). 2014. *Towards a Safer Khayelitsha: Report of the Commission of Inquiry into Allegations of Police Inefficiency and a Breakdown in Relations between SAPS and the Community of Khayelitsha*. Cape Town: KCOI.

Kleinman, Arthur. 1988. *The Illness Narratives: Suffering, Healing, and the Human Condition*. New York: Basic Books.

Knight, Kelly Ray. 2015. *Addicted. Pregnant. Poor*. Durham, NC: Duke University Press.

Koch, Erin. 2016. "Negotiating 'The Social' and Managing Tuberculosis in Georgia." *Journal of Bioethical Inquiry* 13 (1): 47–55. https://doi.org/10.1007/s11673-015-9689-6.

Leonhardt, Kathryn Kraft, Felicia Gentile, Bradley P. Gilbert, and Mary Aiken. 1994. "A Cluster of Tuberculosis among Crack House Contacts in San Mateo County, California." *American Journal of Public Health* 84 (11): 1834–1835.

Leshner, Alan I. 1997. "Addition Is a Brain Disease, and It Matters." *Science* 278 (5335): 45–47. https://doi.org/10.1126/science.278.5335.45.

Lewin, Simon, and Judith Green. 2009. "Ritual and the Organisation of Care in Primary Care Clinics in Cape Town, South Africa." *Social Science & Medicine* 68 (8): 1464–1471. https://doi.org/10.1016/j.socscimed.2009.02.013.

Livingston, Julie. 2012. *Improvising Medicine: An African Oncology Ward in an Emerging Cancer Epidemic*. Durham, NC: Duke University Press.

London, L. 2009. "Confinement for Extensively Drug-Resistant Tuberculosis: Balancing Protection of Health Systems, Individual Rights and the Public's Health." *International Journal of Tuberculosis and Lung Disease* 13 (10): 1200–1209.

London, Leslie. 1999. "The 'Dop' System, Alcohol Abuse and Social Control amongst Farm Workers in South Africa: A Public Health Challenge." *Social Science and Medicine* 48 (10): 1407–1414. https://doi.org/10.1016/S0277-9536(98)00445-6.

Louw, J. H. 1979. "A Brief History of the Medical Faculty, University of Cape Town." *South African Medical Journal* 56 (22): 864–870.

Lovell, Anne M. 2013. "Elusive Travelers: Russian Narcology, Transnational Toxicomanias, and the Great French Ecoholical Experiment." In *Addiction Trajectories*, edited by Eugene Raikhel and William Garriott, 126–159. Durham, NC: Duke University Press.

Macdonald, Helen. 2020. "Using local statistics to tinker with TB treatment in a central Indian clinic." In *Understanding Tuberculosis and Its Control: Anthropological and Ethnographic Approaches*, edited by Helen Macdonald and Ian Harper, 106–125. London: Routledge.

Macdonald, Helen, Paul Mason, and Ian Harper. 2019. "Introduction: Persistent Pathogen." In *Understanding Tuberculosis and Its Control: Anthropological and Ethnographic Approaches*, edited by Helen MacDonald and Ian Harper. London: Routledge.

Maher, Lisa. 2002. "Don't Leave Us This Way: Ethnography and Injecting Drug Use in the Age of AIDS." *International Journal of Drug Policy* 9: 311–325.

Mahon, Rianne, and Fiona Robinson, eds. 2011. *Feminist Ethics and Social Policy: Towards a New Global Political Economy of Care.* Vancouver: UBC Press.

Mail and Guardian. 2009. "'Dumping Ground' for Unwanted People," 9 October. https://mg .co.za/article/2009-10-09-dumping-ground-for-unwanted-people/.

Malotte, Kevin, Fen Rhodes, and Kathleen Mais. 1998. "Tuberculosis Screening and Compliance with Return for Skin Test Reading among Active Drug Users." *American Journal of Public Health* 88 (5): 792–796.

Manasa, Justen, David Katzenstein, Sharon Cassol, Marie-Louise Newell, and Tulio de Oliveira, for the Southern Africa Treatment and Resistance Network. 2012. "Primary Drug Resistance in South Africa: Data from 10 Years of Surveys." *AIDS Research and Human Retroviruses* 28 (6): 558–565.

Marks, Shula. 2006. "The Silent Scourge? Silicosis, Respiratory Disease and Gold-Mining in South Africa." *Journal of Ethnic and Migration Studies* 32 (4): 569–589.

Marlatt, G. Alan. 1996. "Harm Reduction: Come as You Are." *Addictive Behaviours* 21 (6): 779–788. https://doi.org/10.1016/0306-4603(96)00042-1.

Mattingly, Cheryl. 2014. *Moral Laboratories: Family Peril and the Struggle for a Good Life.* Berkeley: University of California Press.

May, Philip A., Jason Blankenship, Anna Susan Marais, J. Phillip Gossage, Wendy O. Kalberg, Ronel Barnard, Marlene De Vries, et al. 2013. "Approaching the Prevalence of the Full Spectrum of Fetal Alcohol Spectrum Disorders in a South African Population-Based Study." *Alcoholism: Clinical and Experimental Research* 37 (5): 818–830. https://doi.org/10 .1111/acer.12033.

May, Philip A., Lesley J. Brooke, Philip J Gossage, Julie Croxford, Colleen Adnams, Kenneth L. Jones, Luther Robinson, and Denis Viljoen. 2000. "Epidemiology of Fetal Alcohol Syndrome in a South African Community in the Western Cape Province." *American Journal of Public Health* 90 (12): 1905–1912. https://doi.org/10.2105/AJPH.90.12.1905.

Mbembe, Achille. 2003. "Necropolitics." *Public Culture* 15 (1): 11–40. https://doi.org/10.1215 /08992363-15-1-11.

Meyers, Todd. 2013. *The Clinic and Elsewhere: Addiction, Adolescents, and the Afterlife of Therapy.* Seattle: University of Washington Press.

Miller, William R., Verner S. Westerberg, Richard J. Harris, and J. Scott Tonigan. 1996. "What Predicts Relapse? Prospective Testing of Antecedent Models." *Addiction* 91 (Suppl.): S155–S171.

Mkhwanazi, Nolwazi. 2016. "Medical Anthropology in Africa: The Trouble with a Single Story." *Medical Anthropology: Cross Cultural Studies in Health and Illness* 35 (2): 193–202. https:// doi.org/10.1080/01459740.2015.1100612.

Mol, Annemarie, Ingunn Moser, and Jeannette Pols, eds. 2010. *Care in Practice: On Tinkering in Clinics, Homes and Farms.* Piscataway, NJ: Transaction Publishers.

Monaghan, Geoffrey, and Dave Bewley-Taylor. 2013. "Police Support for Harm Reduction Policies and Practices towards People Who Inject Drugs." In *Modernising Drug Law Enforcement: Report 1.* London: International Drug Policy Consortium. http://fileserver .idpc.net/library/MDLE-report-1_Police-support-for-harm-reduction.pdf.

Moore, David. 1993. "Ethnography and Illicit Drug Use: Dispatches from an Anthropologist in the 'Field.'" *Addiction Research & Theory* 1: 11–25. https://doi.org/10.3109/16066359309035320.

Moore, David, and Suzanne Fraser. 2006. "Putting at Risk What We Know: Reflecting on the Drug-Using Subject in Harm Reduction and Its Political Implications." *Social Science and Medicine* 62 (12): 3035–3047. https://doi.org/10.1016/j.socscimed.2005.11.067.

Morozova, Olga, Sergii Dvoryak, and Frederick L. Altice. 2013. "Methadone Treatment Improves Tuberculosis Treatment among Hospitalized Opioid Dependent Patients in

Ukraine." *International Journal of Drug Policy* 24 (6): 91–98. https://doi.org/10.1016/j .drugpo.2013.09.001.

Nattrass, Nicoli. 2007. *Mortal Combat: AIDS Denialism and the Struggle for Antiretrovirals in South Africa.* Durban: University of KwaZulu-Natal Press.

Naude, Jim te Water, Leslie London, Blanche Pitt, and Carol Mohamed. 2003. "The 'Dop' System around Stellenbosch—Results from a Farm Survey." *Journal of Southern African Studies* 29 (3): 657–680. https://doi.org/10.1080/0305707032000094965.

Oeltmann, John E., J. Steve Kammerer, Eric S. Pevzner, and Patrick K. Moonan. 2009. "Tuberculosis and Substance Abuse in the United States, 1997–2006." *Archives of Internal Medicine* 169 (2): 189–197. https://doi.org/10.1001/archinternmed.2008.535.

Office of the Premier of the Province of the Western Cape. 2008. "Western Cape Liquor Act." *Provincial Gazette Extraordinary,* 27 November.

Packard, Randall. 1989. *White Plague, Black Labor: Tuberculosis and the Political Economy of Health and Disease in South Africa.* Berkeley: University of California Press.

Packard, Randall, and Paul Epstein. 1991. "Epidemiologists, Social Scientists, and the Structure of Medical Research on Aids in Africa." *Social Science and Medicine* 33 (7): 771–783. https://doi.org/10.1016/0277-9536(91)90376-N.

Pasche, Sonja, and Bronwyn Myers. 2012. "Substance Misuse Trends in South Africa." *Human Psychopharmacology: Clinical and Experimental* 27 (3): 338–341. https://doi.org/10.1002/hup.2228.

Paterson, Craig. 2009. "Prohibition and Resistance: A Socio-Political Exploration of the Changing Dynamics of the Southern African Cannabis Trade, c.1850—the Present." Master's thesis, Rhodes University.

Peltzer, Karl, Julia Louw, Gugu Mchunu, Pamela Naidoo, Gladys Matseke, and Bomkazi Tutshana. 2012. "Hazardous and Harmful Alcohol Use and Associated Factors in Tuberculosis Public Primary Care Patients in South Africa." *International Journal of Environmental Research and Public Health* 9 (9): 3245–3257. https://doi.org/10.3390/ijerph9093245.

Petersen, Zaino, Bronwyn Myers, Marie-Claire van Hout, Andreas Plüddemann, and Charles Parry. 2013. "Availability of HIV Prevention and Treatment Services for People Who Inject Drugs: Findings from 21 Countries." *Harm Reduction Journal* 10 (1): 1–7. https://doi.org /10.1186/1477-7517-10-13.

Petryna, Adriana. 2013. *Life Exposed.* Princeton, NJ: Princeton University Press.

Pienaar, Kiran, and Michael Savic. 2015. "Producing Alcohol and Other Drugs as a Policy 'Problem': A Critical Analysis of South Africa's 'National Drug Master Plan' (2013–2017)." *International Journal of Drug Policy* 30 (2016): 35–42. https://doi.org/10.1016/j.drugpo.2015.12.013.

Pinnock, Don. 2016. *Gang Town.* Cape Town: Tafelberg.

Platsky, Lauren, and Cheryl Walker. 1985. *The Surplus People: Forced Removals in South Africa.* Johannesburg: Raven Press.

Porter, Theodore M. 1996. *Trust in Numbers: The Pursuit of Objectivity in Science and Public Life.* Princeton, NJ: Princeton University Press.

———. 2012. "Funny Numbers." *Culture Unbound* 4: 585–598.

Posel, Deborah. 2001. "Race as Common Sense: Racial Classification in Twentieth-Century South Africa." *African Studies Review* 44 (2): 87–114. https://doi.org/10.2307/525576.

Power, Robert. 2002. "The Application of Ethnography, with Reference to Harm Reduction in Sverdlovk Russia." *International Journal of Drug Policy* 13: 327–331.

Ransome, Arthur. 1898. "Sanatoria for the Open-Air Treatment of Consumption." *British Medical Journal,* July 9: 69–73.

Republic of South Africa. 2004. *The South African National Tuberculosis Control Programme: Practical Guidelines.* Pretoria: National Department of Health. http://www.kznhealth.gov .za/tbguidelines.pdf.

————. 2013. *Management of Drug-Resistant TB: Policy Guidelines*. Pretoria: National Department of Health. https://www.tbonline.info/media/uploads/documents/guidelines_for_management_of_drug-resistant_tuberculosis_in_south_africa_%282013%29.compressed.pdf.

————. 2014. *National Tuberculosis Management Guidelines*. Pretoria: National Department of Health. http://www.kznhealth.gov.za/family/NTCP_Adult_TB_Guidelines_2014.pdf.

Ross, Fiona C. 2010. *Raw Life, New Hope: Decency, Housing and Everyday Life in a Post-Apartheid Community*. Cape Town: University of Cape Town Press.

Rothman, Sheila M. 1995. *Living in the Shadow of Death: Tuberculosis and the Social Experience of Illness in American History*. Baltimore: Johns Hopkins University Press.

Sangaramoorthy, T., and A. Benton. 2021. "Intersectionality and Syndemics: A Commentary." *Social Science and Medicine* 295: 113783. https://doi.org/10.1016/j.socscimed.2021.113783.

Saris, Jamie. 2013. "Committed to Will: What's at Stake for Anthropology." In *Addiction Trajectories*, edited by Eugene Raikhel and William Garriott, 263–283. Durham, NC: Duke University Press.

Scheibe, Andrew, Shaun Shelly, and Anna Versfeld. 2020. "Prohibitionist Drug Policy in South Africa—Reasons and Effects." In *Drug Policies and Development: Conflict and Coexistence*, edited by Julia Buxton, Mary Chinery-Hess, and Khalid Tinasti, 274–304. Geneva: Graduate Institute of International and Development Studies. https://doi.org/10.1163/9789004440494.

Scheibe, Andrew, Shaun Shelly, Anna Versfeld, Simon Howell, and Monique Marks. 2017. "Safe Treatment and Treatment of Safety: Call for a Harm-Reduction Approach to Drug-Use Disorders in South Africa." *South African Health Review* 1: 197–204.

Scheibe, Andrew, Shaun Shelly, and Janine Wildschut. 2018. "Empathic Response and No Need for Perfection: Reflections on Harm Reduction Engagement in South Africa." *Critical Public Health* 1596: 1–11. https://doi.org/10.1080/09581596.2018.1443204.

Scheper-Hughes, Nancy. 1993. "AIDS, Public Health and Human Rights in Cuba." *Lancet* 342 (8877): 965–967. https://doi.org/10.1016/0140-6736(93)92006-f.

Schnippel, K., N. Ndjeka, G. Maartens, G. Meintjes, I. Master, N. Ismail, J. Hughes, et al. 2018. "Effect of Bedaquiline on Mortality in South African Patients with Drug-Resistant Tuberculosis—Authors' Reply." *The Lancet Respiratory Medicine* 6 (12): e57. https://doi.org/10.1016/S2213-2600(18)30451-X.

Schnippel, Kathryn, Sydney Rosen, Kate Shearer, Neil Martinson, Lawrence Long, and Ian Sanne. 2013. "Costs of Inpatient Treatment for Multi-Drug-Resistant Tuberculosis in South Africa." *Tropical Medicine and International Health* 18 (1): 109–116. https://doi.org/10.1111/tmi.12018.

Schoeman, Willem J. 2017. "South African Religious Demography: The 2013 General Household Survey." *HTS Teologiese Studies/Theological Studies* 73 (2): 1–7. https://doi.org/10.4102/hts.v73i2.3837.

Schüll, Natasha Dow. 2013. "Balancing Acts: Gambling-Machine Addiction." In *Addiction Trajectories*, edited by Eugene Raikhel and William Garriott, 61–87. Durham, NC: Duke University Press.

Seeberg, Jens. 2013a. "The Death of Shankar: Social Exclusion and Tuberculosis in a Poor Neighbourhood in Bhubaneswar, Odisha." In *Navigating Social Exclusion and Inclusion in Contemporary India and Beyond: Structures, Agents, Practices*, edited by Uwe Skoda, Kenneth Bo Nielsen, and Marianne Qvortrup Fibiger, 207–226. London: Anthem Press.

————. 2013b. "The Death of Shankar: Tuberculosis and Social Exclusion in a Poor Neighbourhood in Bhubaneswar, Odisha." In *Navigating Social Exclusion and Inclusion in Contemporary India and Beyond*, edited by Uwe Skoda, Kenneth Nielsen, and Marianne Qvortrup Sudoka, 207–226. London: Anthem.

Setswe, G., A. Cloete, M. Mabaso, S. Jooste, Y. Ntsepe, S. Mswelli, S. Sigida, and R. Molobeli. 2015. "Programmatic Mapping and Size Estimation Study of Key Populations in South Africa: Sex Workers (Male and Female), Men Who Have Sex with Men, Persons Who Inject Drugs and Transgender People." Cape Town: NACOSA.

Simangan, Dahlia. 2018. "Is the Philippine 'War on Drugs' an Act of Genocide?" *Journal of Genocide Research* 20 (1): 68–89. https://doi.org/10.1080/14623528.2017.1379939.

Singer, Merrill. 2000. "A Dose of Drugs, a Touch of Violence, a Case of AIDS: Conceptualizing the SAVA Syndemic." *Free Inquiry in Creative Sociology* 28 (1): 13–24.

———. 2006. "A Dose of Drugs, a Touch of Violence, a Case of AIDS: Further Conceptualizing the SAVA Syndemic." *Free Inquiry in Creative Sociology* 34 (1): 39–54.

———. 2009. *Introduction to Syndemics: A Critical Systems Approach to Public and Community Health*. San Francisco: John Wiley & Sons.

———. 2012. "Anthropology and Addiction: An Historical Review." *Addiction* 107 (10): 1747–1755. https://doi.org/10.1111/j.1360-0443.2012.03879.x.

———. 2014. "The Infectious Disease Syndemics of Crack Cocaine." *Journal of Equity in Health* 3 (1): 32–44.

Singer, Merrill, Nicola Bulled, and Bayla Ostrach. 2020. "Whither Syndemics? Trends in Syndemics Research, a Review 2015–2019." *Global Public Health* 15 (7): 943–955. https://doi.org/10.1080/17441692.2020.1724317.

Singer, Merrill, Nicola Bulled, Bayla Ostrach, and Emily Mendenhall. 2017. "Syndemics and the Biosocial Conception of Health." *The Lancet* 389 (10072): 941–950. https://doi.org/10.1016/S0140-6736(17)30003-X.

Singer, Merrill, and Scott Clair. 2003. "Syndemics and Public Health: Reconceptualizing Disease in Bio-Social Context." *Medical Anthropology Quarterly* 17 (4): 423–441.

Singer, Merrill, Freddie Valentin, Hans Baer, and Zhongke Jia. 1992. "Why Does Juan Garcia Have a Drinking Problem? The Perspective of Critical Medical Anthropology." *Medical Anthropology* 14 (1): 77–108.

Singh, Jerome Amir, Ross Upshur, and Nesri Padayatchi. 2007. "XDR-TB in South Africa: No Time for Denial or Complacency." *PLoS Medicine* 4 (1): 0019–0025. https://doi.org/10.1371/journal.pmed.0040050.

Standing, Andre. 2006. *Organised Crime on the Cape Flats*. Pretoria: Institute of Security Studies.

Statistics South Africa. 2013. "Statistical Release P0302: Mid-Year Population Estimates 2013." Pretoria: Statistics South Africa. https://doi.org/Statistical release P0302.

Stein Dan and Manyedi Eva, for the Executive Committee of the Central Drug Authority. 2016. "Position Statement on Cannabis: A Step Forwards." *South African Medical Journal* 106 (9): 837.

Stevenson, Lisa. 2014. *Life Beside Itself: Imagining Care in the Canadian Arctic*. San Francisco: University of California Press.

Stillo, Jonathan. 2015. "We Are the Losers of Socialism." *Anthropological Journal of European Cultures* 24 (1): 132–140.

Street, Alice. 2014. *Biomedicine in an Unstable Place: Infrastructure and Personhood in a Papua New Guinean Hospital*. Durham, NC: Duke University Press.

Tate, Winifred. 2015. *Drugs, Thugs, and Diplomats: US Policymaking in Colombia*. Stanford, CA: Stanford University Press.

Ticktin, Miriam. 2006. "Where Ethics and Politics Meet: The Violence of Humanitarianism in France." *American Ethnologist* 33 (1): 33–49.

Vale, Beth, Rebecca Hodes, Lucie Cluver, and Mildred Thabeng. 2017. "Bureaucracies of Blood and Belonging: Documents, HIV-Positive Youth and the State in South Africa." *Development and Change* 48 (313421): 1287–1309. https://doi.org/10.1111/dech.12341.

van der Geest, Sjaak, and Kaja Finkler. 2004. "Hospital Ethnography: Introduction." *Social Science and Medicine* 59: 1995–2001. https://doi.org/10.1016/j.socscimed.2004.03.004.

van der Vliet, Virginia. 2007. "Ruined Dreams? Confronting AIDS in South Africa." *Conflict, Security & Development* 7 (2): 349–359. https://doi.org/10.1080/14678800701358785.

Van Rensburg, Dingie, Ega Van Rensburg-Bonthuyzen, Christo Heunis, and Herman Meulemans. 2005. "Tuberculosis Control in South Africa: Reasons for Persistent Failure." *Acta Academica Suplementum* 1 (1): 1–55.

Venkat, Bharat Jayram. 2016. "Cures." *Public Culture* 28 (380): 475–497. https://doi.org/10.1215/08992363-3511502.

Versfeld, Anna. 2012a. "All Pay and No Work: Spheres of Belonging under Duress." Unpublished master's thesis. University of Cape Town.

Versfeld, Anna. 2012b. "Generational Change in Manenberg: The Erosion of Possibilities for Positive Personhood." *Agenda* 26 (4): 101–113.

Versfeld, Anna, Angela McBride, Andrew Scheibe and C. Wendy Spearman. 2020. "Motivations, Facilitators and Barriers to Accessing Hepatitis C Treatment among People Who Inject Drugs in Two South African Cities." *Harm Reduction Journal* 17 (1): 1–8. https://doi.org/10.1186/s12954-020-00382-3.

Viljoen, Denis, Phillip Gossage, Lesley Brooke, Colleen Adnams, Kenneth Jones, Luther Robinson, Eugene Hoyme, et al. 2005. "Fetal Alcohol Syndrome Epidemiology in a South African Community: A Second Study of a Very High Prevalence Area." *Journal of Studies on Alcohol* 66 (5): 593–604.

Watermeyer, Laura. 2013. "Drug Use Spirals in Cape but Services Lag Behind." *Cape Times*, 16 October.

Weaver, Lesley Jo, and Emily Mendenhall. 2014. "Applying Syndemics and Chronicity: Interpretations from Studies of Poverty, Depression, and Diabetes." *Medical Anthropology* 33 (2): 92–108. https://doi.org/10.1080/01459740.2013.808637.

Western Cape Government. 2016. *Socio-Economic Profile: City of Cape Town, 2016*. City of Cape Town. https://www.westerncape.gov.za/assets/departments/treasury/Documents/Socio-economic-profiles/2016/City-of-Cape-Town/city_of_cape_town_2016_socio-economic_profile_sep-lg.pdf.

Western Cape Government. 2017. *Socio-Economic Profile: City of Cape Town 2017*. City of Cape Town. https://www.westerncape.gov.za/assets/departments/treasury/Documents/Socio-economic-profiles/2017/city_of_cape_town_2017_socio-economic_profile_sep-lg_-_26_january_2018.pdf.

Wilby, K. J., M. H. Ensom, and F. Marra. 2014. "Review of Evidence for Measuring Drug Concentrations of First-Line Antitubercular Agents in Adults." *Clinical Pharmacokinetics* 53 (10): 873–890.

Williams, Theodore C. 1876. "Lettsomian Lectures on the Influence of Climate on the Treatment of Pulmonary Consumption." *British Medical Journal*, 8 January, 38–42.

World Health Organization. 1983. *Apartheid and Health*. Geneva: World Health Organization.

———2006. *Guidelines for the Programmatic Management of Drug-Resistant Tuberculosis*. Geneva: World Health Organization.

———. 2008. *Policy Guidelines for Collaborative TB and HIV Services for Injecting and Other Drug Users*. Geneva: World Health Organization.

———. 2013. *Global Tuberculosis Report 2013*. Geneva: World Health Organization.

———. 2016. *Global Tuberculosis Report 2016*. Geneva: World Health Organization.

———. 2018. *Global Tuberculosis Report 2018*. Geneva: World Health Organization.

World Health Organization, United Nations Office on Drugs and Crime, and UNAIDS. 2008. *Policy Guidelines for Collaborative TB and HIV Services for Injecting and Other Drug Users:*

An Integrated Approach. Geneva: World Health Organization. http://apps.who.int/iris
/bitstream/handle/10665/43937/9789241596930_eng.pdf;jsessionid=8AA5200CE96952
CCD46D178D274AF5F2?sequence=1.

Zigon, Jarrett. 2010. "'A Disease of Frozen Feelings.'" *Medical Anthropology Quarterly* 24 (3):
326–343. https://doi.org/10.1111/j.1548-1387.2010.01107.x.

Zumla, Alimuddin, Payam Nahid, and Stewart T. Cole. 2013. "Advances in the Development
of New Tuberculosis Drugs and Treatment Regimens." *Nature Reviews Drug Discovery*
12 (4): 388–404. https://doi.org/10.1038/nrd4001.

INDEX

abstinence, 19, 30–32, 37, 56, 85, 106, 108;
    binary between substance use and, 24,
    40–41, 65–66, 103, 108–109, 114–115
Adams, Vincanne, 63, 70, 130n18
addiction, 21–22, 40, 66, 107, 109–110, 119; and
    assumptions of inevitable relapse, 30, 34,
    108, 115; disease model of, 31–33, 35, 40, 108,
    119; language of, 78; and "Rat Park"
    experiment, 34–35
African/Black, 6, 10, 22
African National Congress (ANC) government,
    12–13
African Union, 38–39
Alcoholics or Narcotics Anonymous (AA/NA),
    30–31. *See also* occupational therapy
    awareness sessions, DP Marais: AA
    "name and shame" philosophy of
alcohol use, 2, 10, 21, 40, 48–49, 55, 64, 103, 116,
    127n13; anthropological inputs on, 33; and
    dop system, 8, 127n11; and fetal alcohol
    syndrome (FAS), 8, 36, 47, 95, 129n7, 132n9.
    See also substance use; treatment default:
    substance use as risk factor for
Alexander, Bruce, 35. *See also* addiction: and
    "Rat Park" experiment
anthropological approaches to substance use,
    24–25, 33–34; critical medical, 33. *See also*
    experiential model anthropology
anthropology in action, 25, 120
antiretrovirals (ARV). *See* antiretroviral
    therapy (ART)
antiretroviral therapy (ART), 12–13, 16–17, 43,
    47, 74, 97, 128n22; and alleged smoking of
    ARVs, 83; second-line, 97, 132n14
apartheid, 6, 10, 12, 48; education system, 86;
    homelands, 46–47, 129n4; structural effects
    of, 6–7, 23. *See also* Group Areas Act of
    1951; mandrax: apartheid state's relation-
    ship with

Bacille Calmette-Guérin (BCG) vaccine, 52,
    130n16
"Bantustans." *See* apartheid: homelands

Bateman, Chris, 14–15, 27
bedaquiline, 15–16
biomedical approach to disease, 17, 50;
    limitations of, 4–5, 52–55, 57, 76, 101.
    See also syndemics
Biruk, Crystal, 61, 71
blame, 3, 32, 34–36, 47, 57; and narratives
    of self-accountability, 46, 49, 85–88. *See also*
    occupational therapy awareness sessions,
    DP Marais: AA "name and shame"
    philosophy of
Bourgois, Philippe, 33–34

cannabis use, 2, 7–10, 29; regulation of, 8.
    See also dagga
Cape Flats, 6–7, 10
care provision, 17, 24–25; and broader needs
    of families, 95, 98–99; and concept of
    "good" care, 84, 94–95, 100; implications
    of co-constitution for, 54, 57, 100–101;
    improvization as characteristic of, 17, 101;
    patient ambivalence about, 97–99; and
    providers' involvement in departure/
    discharge planning, 103–106, 112, 114;
    rights-based, 24, 84; "tinkering" in, 53,
    83–84, 132n1
Carr, Summerson, 19, 30–31, 34
Central Drug Authority. *See* Department of
    Social Development
cigarettes, 31, 44, 64, 88–89, 96, 110, 127n10,
    130n3
City of Cape Town, 1–2, 8–9, 47; anti-
    substance use campaign in, 27–28, 31;
    colonial/apartheid history of, 6–7;
    landscape of TB in, 15, 17, 23, 49; private
    treatment center industry in, 28. *See also*
    Delft; DP Marais TB Hospital, Cape
    Town; Manenberg, Cape Town
Clair, Scott, 5, 55
co-constitution. *See* substance use–TB
    co-constitution
Coloured, 10, 22, 127n7
Constitutional Court, 8

147

TB (Tuberculosis) cure, 74–75; individual
responsibility for, 73–74, 78, 82, 84; statistics
for drug-sensitive TB, 3, 14, 127n3, 127n19
TB diagnosis and treatment: difficulties
associated with, 49–51, 53, 129n12;
GeneXpert technology, 49, 129nn9–10;
and limitations of standardized treatment,
82–83; and prophylactics, 77, 79; substance
use as complicating factor in, 5, 51–52
TB epidemic, 9; historical miscasting of black
bodies in, 11–13; impact of incarceration
on, 2; incident rates in South Africa, 3, 13;
as leading cause of deaths, 3, 127n4, 129n15;
nosocomial spread of, 15, 94
TB/HIV Care Association, 79, 121; Step Up
Project, 26–27, 70–71, 128n1
TB meningitis, 50–51, 97, 132n12
TB–substance use intersection, 2–3, 5, 7, 19,
22–23, 110. See also substance use–TB
co-constitution
tertiary care hospitals, 1, 17, 43, 68–69, 80, 96,
127n2
tik, 7, 51, 55, 62, 106–107; biochemical effects
of, 9–10, 56; as "drug of choice," 9, 127n13;
interaction between TB and, 63–64, 69, 80,
96, 108–109; withdrawal symptoms, 50, 93.
See also methamphetamine
tobacco. See cigarettes
treatment adherence, 13, 24, 40, 120
treatment default, 1–2, 42–43, 45, 87–89, 91,
127n1; substance use as risk factor for, 3,
72–73, 92. See also treatment interruption;
"unruly" patients: treatment default by
treatment interruption, 2, 22, 24, 127n1;
consequences of, 75, 87; link between
substance use and, 3, 40–42, 56, 90, 117.
See also treatment default

treatment nonadherence. See treatment
default
Truth and Reconciliation Commission,
South Africa, 8–9

United Kingdom, 28, 38
United Nations General Assembly
(UNGASS), 38
"unruly" patients, 72, 113; binary tropes of
"good" and, 76, 81, 98, 109, 118, 121; DP
Marais as place of containment for, 73–76,
80; impact on family and household
members, 73, 75–79; impact on recordkeeping processes, 75–76; the making of,
79; treatment default by, 72–73, 77–78, 118;
undermining of health care providers by,
75–76, 131n2

Venkat, Bharat, 63, 127n19
violence, 4, 54, 78, 84; gang, 7; sexual, 10, 99;
structural, 119. See also syndemics: SAVA

weekend/day passes, 89–90; denial of,
91–93
Western Cape Province, 3, 13; shift away from
DOTS, 14, 127n15; winelands, 8
White, 6, 10, 23
Whiteness, 22
women: appeal of tik for, 10, 64; and ART,
12; community health work and, 14; and
stigma of substance abuse, 28; vulnerability
of young, 113. See also gender discrimination
World Health Organization (WHO), 2–3, 13,
15, 37, 120; definition of harm reduction
interventions, 39; Global Tuberculosis
Report, 59, 127n3; guidelines for managing
TB, 39–40

ABOUT THE AUTHOR

ANNA VERSFELD is an independent South African medical anthropologist and an honorary research affiliate in the Department of Social Anthropology at the University of Cape Town. She consults globally on social dynamics of tuberculosis, vulnerable populations, and people-centered health care provision. Within this work she holds a commitment to health equity and inclusive social research.

Available titles in the Medical Anthropology:
Health, Inequality, and Social Justice series